Persistent Cough, Chronic Cough and Dry Cough

What you need to know about the causes and treatments of Persistent Cough, Chronic Cough and Dry Cough

Persistent Cough, Chronic Cough and Dry Cough

What you need to know about the causes and treatments of Persistent Cough, Chronic Cough and Dry Cough

BY

Daniel Levin

Mechiel Publishing

The ideas, information and suggestions in this book are purely the ideas of the author and are not substitutes for consulting your physician. We will not accept responsibility for any action or claim resulting from the use of information contained in this book.

First published in 2017 by Mechiel Publishing

Copyright © Mechiel Publishing 2017

Persistent Cough, Chronic Cough and Dry Cough

Foreword

We are all familiar with that annoying tickle in our throats – the kind that signals an oncoming cold. Most of the time, this unpleasant symptom only sticks around for a few days, but some people suffer from persistent or chronic cough that lasts for weeks, or even months. But what prevents your body from kicking the cough and why do some people seem to be more susceptible to coughs and colds than others?

Chronic or persistent cough can be the result of many potential causes and it may produce different symptoms in different people. Perhaps you have a stuffed-up or runny nose, or maybe you feel a constant drip of liquid down the back of your throat. Maybe you find yourself clearing your throat every ten minutes or your throat feels dry and your voice is hoarse. These are just a few of the many symptoms which can accompany a chronic cough or dry cough and they can cause an impairment in your ability to sleep, eat, or even enjoy your day.

If you or a loved one suffers from chronic cough or persistent dry cough, it is not something that you should ignore – especially if it has been going on for more than a week or two. In this book, you will learn how to tell the difference between a regular cold and a case of chronic cough or dry cough. You will learn about the various symptoms as well as the potential causes. By the time you finish this book you will have a better understanding of this common health problem, as well as how to deal with it both medically and naturally.

So, if you are ready to say goodbye to your chronic cough, simply turn the page and keep reading!

Table of Contents

Introduction

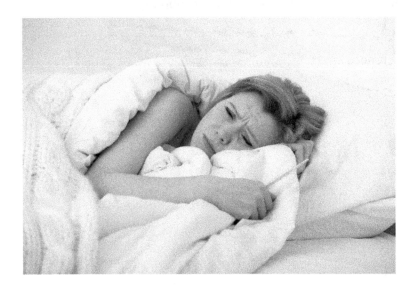

When you feel that telltale tickle in your throat, you know that a cough is coming on. But what kind of cough will it be? Is it the kind of cough that will come and go in less than a week, or will it linger for a month or more? Many people do not understand the difference between acute cough and chronic cough, but you will learn the difference very quickly if it ever happens to you. Having a cough that lasts for weeks and weeks is by no means pleasant and it is not something you'll soon forget.

In this book, you will learn everything you have ever wanted to know (and more) about coughs. You'll be introduced to the six most common types of cough and take a deeper look into the differences between dry cough vs. wet cough and acute cough vs. chronic cough. You are going to learn some interesting facts and statistics about the different coughs and their causes, plus you'll explore the most common remedies for colds and coughs – both medicinal and natural. You'll even receive a collection of cough-busting recipes.

By the time you finish this book, all of your questions about dry cough and chronic cough will be answered and the next time you feel a tickle in your throat, you will be prepared. So, what are you waiting for? Turn the page and keep reading!

Chapter 1: Types of Cough and What They Mean

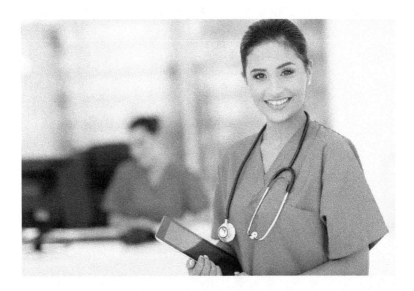

A cough is a cough – right? Not necessarily. Many people do not realize that a cough isn't the same thing as a cold – it is a symptom that can be associated with a wide variety of different things. A cough is simply a mechanism your body uses to clear your airway of some kind of blockage – it may also be an involuntary response to irritation in your throat.

When you cough, it clears your throat of mucus (or postnasal drip) and it helps to open up your windpipe so more air can flow through. Though coughs can be caused by a number of different things, there are technically two types of coughs – productive coughs and unproductive coughs. A productive cough is one that produces phlegm or mucus. An unproductive cough is one that does not produce mucus – it is sometimes called a "dry" cough for this reason.

Now that you understand the two different types of coughs, you can better understand the various causes. In the following pages, you will receive an overview of the six most common types of cough including symptoms and causes.

1. Asthma

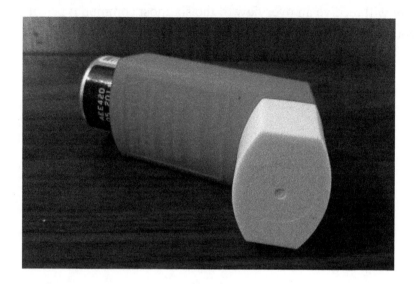

Asthma is a condition that affects the lungs and it can cause chest tightness, wheezing, and coughing. Individuals who suffer from asthma may experience narrowing or swelling of the airways which causes the chest to feel tight – they may also develop excess mucus which can impair breathing and trigger episodes of coughing. Many people who suffer from asthma find that their cough is worst in the morning and at night. Unfortunately, asthma cannot be cured but there are various methods for control.

The symptoms of asthma may vary from one person to another and they may also vary in severity. The most common symptoms include the following:

- Shortness of breath
- Chest pain or tightness
- Coughing and wheezing
- Whistling sound upon exhale

- Attacks worsened by a respiratory virus

For many people asthma is mild and doesn't have a significant impact on their daily lives. For others, however, severe asthma attacks can be triggered by exercise, environmental irritants, or allergies. <u>The underlying cause for asthma is unknown, but there are a number of different triggers that may include the following</u>:

- Airborne irritants (pet dander, dust mites, pollen, mold, etc.)
- Physical activity (known as exercise-induced asthma)
- Respiratory infection (such as a cold or flu)
- Air pollutants (smoke, perfumes, etc.)
- Certain medications (like aspirin and ibuprofen)
- Sulfites and preservatives in some food
- Gastroesophageal reflux disease (known as GERD)
- Cold air or changes in weather

As already mentioned, the underlying cause for asthma is unknown but there are certain things that can increase your risk. Having a family member with asthma, for example, or having allergies, smoking, being overweight, and working with chemicals can increase your risk. The treatment for asthma usually involves medication such as inhaled corticosteroids and oral medications. You may also need allergy medicine like antihistamines if your asthma is triggered by allergies.

2. COPD

Chronic obstructive pulmonary disease, or COPD, is most frequently caused by smoking. COPD is technically a group of diseases that are characterized by breathing-related problems including airflow blockage. Under the heading of COPD are conditions like emphysema, chronic bronchitis, and even asthma. Though smoking is the number-one cause for COPD, it can also be caused by air pollutants in the home or work place and influenced by genetic factors and respiratory infections.

Emphysema is a disease that is caused by destruction of the alveoli in the bronchioles in the lungs, generally due to cigarette smoke and other irritating gases. Chronic bronchitis is caused by inflammation in the lining of the bronchial tubes which help to carry air to and from the alveoli. Both of these conditions may result in a chronic cough that produces an excess of mucus. This cough tends to be most severe in the morning and it may get better throughout the day. Other symptoms include the following:

- Wheezing
- Chest tightness
- Fatigue
- Shortness of breath
- Excess mucus
- Blue lips or fingernail beds
- Frequent respiratory infection
- Swollen ankles or feet
- Unintended weight loss

Though the most common cause for COPD is cigarette smoke (this includes second-hand smoke), there are certain factors which can increase your risk. <u>Some of the most common risk factors for developing COPD include the following</u>:

- Having asthma (especially combined with smoking)
- Exposure to dust and chemicals at work
- Inhaling fumes from burning fuel (such as cooking)
- Middle age (40 years or older)
- Genetics (especially a condition called alph-1-antitrypsin deficiency)

In addition to a hacking cough, COPD can lead to complications such as frequent respiratory infections, heart problems, lung cancer, high blood pressure, and depression. Stopping smoking is the most important step in treating COPD but certain medications can also be used to manage the symptoms. Some common medications for COPD include bronchodilators, inhaled corticosteroids, oral steroids, and phosphodiesterase-4 inhibitors. Oxygen therapy may also be required and, in severe cases, surgeries like lung volume reduction surgery and lung transplants may be required.

3. GERD

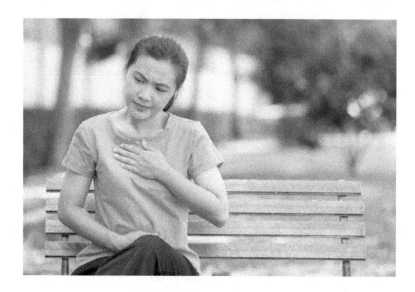

Gastroesophageal reflux disease, or GERD, usually causes a dry cough and it is the second most common cause of dry cough. GERD is a chronic digestive disorder that occurs when your stomach acid (or the contents of the stomach) back up into the esophagus. The acid causes irritation to the lining of the esophagus which leads to acid reflux and heartburn as well as the chronic dry cough. Occasional heartburn is normal, but if symptoms occur more than twice a week or if they begin to affect your day-to-day life, it is time to seek medical attention.

As many as 75% of GERD patients experience chronic cough but no other symptoms. In many cases, the cough worsens when the individual lies down or when he is eating. Other symptoms which may be related to GERD include the following:

- Burning sensation in the chest or throat
- Difficulty swallowing (known as dysphagia)

- Chest pain or tightness
- Chronic dry cough
- Sore throat or hoarseness
- Acid reflux (regurgitation of food or sour liquid)
- Feeling a lump in the throat

The most common cause of GERD is frequent acid reflux. Each time you swallow, the circular band of muscle around the lower part of your esophagus (known as the esophageal sphincter) relaxes so food can flow into the stomach. After swallowing, the opening closes again. In cases of GERD, however, the valve may weaken or relax abnormally which allows stomach acid to flow backward into the esophagus. Over time, this backwash causes irritation to the lining of the esophagus which can also lead to complications such as bleeding or Barrett's esophagus (this is a precancerous condition).

There are certain factors which can increase your risk of developing GERD. Some of the most common risk factors include obesity, pregnancy, smoking, and diabetes. People who have delayed stomach emptying or connective tissue disorders may also be at risk of GERD. Some complications that may be related to GERD include narrowing of the esophagus, esophageal ulcers, and precancerous changes to the esophagus (known as Barrett's esophagus). Treatment generally involves over-the-counter heartburn medications, H-2-receptor blockers, and medications that block acid production and help to heal the esophagus.

4. Pneumonia

Pneumonia is a type of infection that affects the lungs –
particularly the air sacs in the lungs. This disease can be caused
by viruses as well as fungi and bacteria which cause the air sacs in
the lungs to fill with fluid or pus. This causes the patient to
experience a persistent wet cough as well as fever, chills, and
breathing difficulties. The severity of this condition can vary from
mild to life-threatening, though it is generally the most dangerous
for infants, young children, and individuals over the age of 65 – it
is also dangerous for people with impaired immunity and other
health problems.

The signs and symptoms of pneumonia can vary greatly from one
person to another and from one case to another. <u>Some of the most
common symptoms of pneumonia include the following</u>:

- Chest pain when breathing
- Confusion, other mental changes
- Productive cough
- Extreme fatigue
- Fever, chills, and/or sweating
- Low body temperature
- Vomiting or diarrhea
- Shortness of breath

In many cases, infants do not show outward signs of pneumonia
but they may appear restless or tired, have trouble breathing, or
develop a fever and cough. There are certain factors which can
increase your risk of developing pneumonia including being
hospitalized, having a chronic disease, smoking, or having a
weakened immune system. Pneumonia can lead to complications
such as bacteria in the bloodstream (known as bacteremia),

breathing problems, fluid in the lungs (known as pleural effusion), and abscesses forming in the lungs.

The diagnosis for pneumonia can generally be made through blood tests and chest x-rays as well as pulse oximetry and a sputum test. For individuals over the age of 65, additional tests like a CT scan and a fluid sample taken from the lungs may be needed. Treatment for pneumonia is typically aimed toward curing the infection and reducing the risk of complications. Some treatment options include antibiotics, cough medicine, fever reducers, and pain relievers. Hospitalization may be required for individuals over 65 as well as cases of decline in kidney function, mental confusion, low blood pressure, rapid breathing, low body temperature and low heart rate.

5. Postnasal Drip

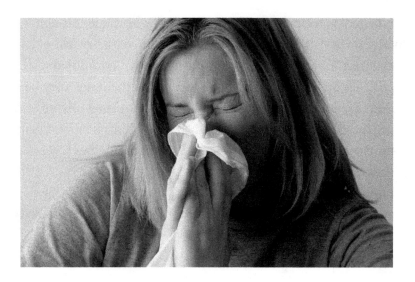

This type of cough is aptly named because it is caused by mucus dripping down the back of your throat. Your body produces mucus every day in the lining of your nose and throat as well as your stomach and intestinal tract. In fact, your nose produces as much as a quart of mucus per day all on its own. Mucus serves an important purpose in the body – it keeps your nose and throat moist while also trapping pathogens and foreign invaders before they cause an infection.

A quart of mucus sounds like a lot. In a way, it is, but you generally don't even notice it. The mucus your nose produces mixes with your saliva and drips down your throat – that is what you are swallowing all day long. It is only when your body starts to produce thicker mucus, or more mucus than usual, that you start to notice it. That is what is happening when you experience postnasal drip.

There are many things that can cause postnasal drip, but some of the more common causes are:

- Cold or flu
- Allergies
- Sinus infections
- Foreign object in the nose
- Certain medications
- Change in weather
- Deviated septum
- Certain foods
- Inhaled irritants

When you have postnasal drip, you may feel a constant desire to clear your throat. The mucus can become thick enough that it starts to block part of your airway, causing you to cough. This kind of cough can be persistent and it often worsens at night. The irritation caused by the excess mucus and all of that coughing can also leave your throat feeling dry and sore.

There are many treatment options for postnasal drip, some of which depend on the cause. For example, if your excess mucus production is due to allergies taking an antihistamine may help. If it's a side effect of a persistent cold, you can try things like inhaling steam or a saline wash to flush away excess mucus and relieve congestion. If the mucus is caused by a bacterial infection, you may need antibiotics to clear it up.

6. Whooping Cough

Also known as pertussis, whooping cough is a severe, hacking cough. Whooping cough is a highly contagious disease and, while a vaccine was developed during the 1940s, it sometimes experiences a resurgence. According to the CDC, nearly 50,000 cases were reported in 2012 which was the highest number since 1955. For the most part, however, whooping cough affects infants and children too young for the vaccination as well as teenagers and adults whose immunity to the disease has worn away.

Though whooping cough is highly contagious, it generally takes 7 to 10 days for symptoms to appear after infection – that is one of the reasons why it is so dangerous. <u>At first, symptoms mimic those of the common cold, including the following</u>:

- Nasal congestion
- Runny nose
- Watery eyes
- Fever
- Persistent cough

After 7 to 14 days, these symptoms may worsen. Mucus in the airways begins to thicken and accumulate, causing uncontrollable coughing. These coughing attacks can become very severe, sometimes becoming so violent that the individual vomits or turns red in the face. After a day or two of violent cough attacks, the individual may also become extremely fatigued and constant strain on the windpipe can produce a high-pitched whooping sound when the individual inhales after a cough.

Whooping cough is generally caused by bacteria and it can be transmitted through the air. In infants under 6 months of age, whooping cough can lead to some serious complications including pneumonia, breathing problems, dehydration, and even seizures or brain damage. Whooping cough can be diagnosed through nose and throat cultures as well as blood samples and chest x-ray. Treatment generally involves antibiotics to kill the bacteria, though there is often little that can be done to relieve the cough itself until the individual recovers.

Any of these six types of coughs can become severe enough to cause serious problems. As a general rule, you should contact your doctor if your cough lasts for more than three weeks or if it continues to worsen over time, instead of getting better. You should also seek medical attention if you begin to have trouble breathing, if you experience chest pain, or if you cough up blood. These things can be signs of a more serious, potentially even life-threatening problem, and should not be ignored.

Now that you understand the six most common types of coughs we are going to explore chronic cough in greater detail. In the next chapter, you will receive some interesting facts and statistics about chronic cough as well as information about the symptoms and causes for this kind of cough.

Chapter 2: Causes of Chronic Cough

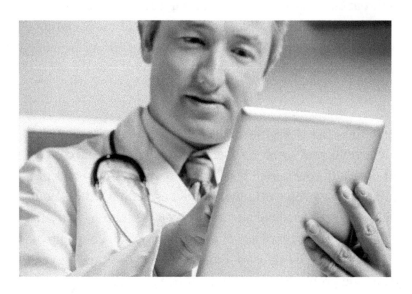

A chronic cough is simply a cough that persists over a long period of time – the qualification is 4 weeks for children and 8 weeks for adults. Chronic cough is not technically a disease or disorder – it is a symptom of an underlying condition. While a cough may be a minor annoyance, chronic cough can eventually become painful and may even cause serious complications like vomiting, light headedness, breathing problems, and rib fractures.

There are many reasons why a cough may not improve and it can sometimes be difficult to identify the exact reason. Once you identify the reason, however, you can treat it and the cough should go away. In this chapter, you'll receive some interesting facts and statistics about chronic cough as well as information about the symptoms and treatments for chronic cough.

1. Facts and Statistics

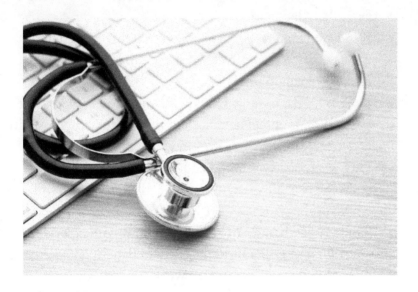

As you have already learned, coughing is an important reflex that the body uses to clear your airway. There are many different conditions which can contribute to chronic cough, and it isn't always easy to identify the one that is to blame. The American College of Chest Physicians (ACCP) analyzed numerous studies and found that the three most common causes for chronic cough are postnasal drip, GERD, and asthma. However, another study showed that the cause of chronic cough goes unidentified in as many as 42% of cases.

You have also learned that there are many different types of coughs – you received detailed information about six of them in the previous chapter. Below you will find some interesting facts and statistics about different types of chronic cough:

- Approximately 30 million Americans are affected by COPD with some states having a prevalence rate as high as 9.1% (Alabama).
- It is estimated that someone dies of COPD in the United States every four minutes – it is the third most common cause of death in the U.S.
- Each year, the cost for COPD treatment totals more than $50 billion in direct healthcare costs and indirect mortality and morbidity costs.
- Each year, nearly 9 million adults are diagnosed with chronic bronchitis (COPD) and nearly 3.5 million with emphysema.
- Approximately 60% of American adults will experience some kind of GERD within a 12-month period and 20% to 30% of those will experience weekly symptoms.
- Women are more likely than men to be hospitalized for GERD symptoms and individuals over the age of 40 account for approximately 50% of diagnosed cases.
- Only 1% of all people diagnosed with GERD develop Barrett's esophagus and it is more common in men, particularly Caucasian men.

At the beginning of this chapter you learned that chronic cough usually lasts for 4 weeks in children and 8 weeks in adults. To give you a better understanding, consider that acute cough (or a short-lived cough) usually resolves within three weeks. The longer chronic cough lasts, the more likely it is to lead to complications. Many people who suffer from chronic cough experience exhaustion and sleep disturbance which can lead to further fatigue. Depending on how severe the cough is, you could also find yourself dealing with other physical complications like rib fractures or pneumothorax (collapsed lung).

The treatment for chronic cough varies according to the cause, but there are many cases where the underlying cause cannot be identified. In cases like this, antitussive therapies may be considered. There are two categories of antitussive therapies – they are divided by the way they act in the body, either centrally or peripherally. Some common centrally acting antitussive therapies include pholcodine, codeine, dextromethorphan, methadone, and morphine. These medications act directly upon the cough center in the brain and lessen the nerve impulse discharges that actually act upon the muscles to produce a cough.

Peripherally acting antitussive therapies work by inhibiting the response of the nerves involved in the cough reflex. Some examples of these agents include humidifying aerosols, demulcents, and local anesthetics. Commonly used local anesthetics include things like benzocaine, lidocaine, tetracaine, and hexylcaine hydrochloride. In cases of nonproductive chronic cough (dry cough), a combined therapy of codeine or dextromethorphan with various expectorants, antihistamines, decongestants, and antipyretics has been found useful.

You will learn more about the most common causes for chronic cough in the next section, but for now you may be interested to learn some of the reasons why a cough may become chronic. Here are some of the top reasons why your cough might not be improving as quickly as you would like:

- Your throat could be irritated following an infection – viral infections can cause swelling and oversensitivity in the airway which can cause your cough to linger.
- Poor sleep quality or lack of sleep can contribute to chronic cough, partially because your body does most of its healing during sleep.

- When you are stressed, it can inhibit your immune response which could not only make you more vulnerable to colds and other infections but which can prevent your body from recovering from cough as quickly as it otherwise would.
- You might not be drinking enough water and other fluids. In addition to hydrating your body, drinking fluids will help to loosen the mucus in your airway so that you can cough it out. Alcoholic drinks and caffeinated beverages can inhibit this.
- You're using too much nasal decongestant spray. When your nose is stuffed up you might turn to a decongestant spray in order to be able to breathe. But if you use these sprays for more than 3 days your symptoms could worsen when you stop and it could cause your cough to stick around longer.
- Breathing in dry air (particularly indoor air) can irritate your throat and exacerbate your cough – use a humidifier or inhale steam if that's your only option. It is best to have an indoor humidity level of 40% to 50%.
- You might be dealing with a secondary bacterial infection as a side effect of a cold. When your airway becomes raw and irritated from a cold it makes it more susceptible to bacteria which can lead to secondary sinus infections, bronchitis, or even pneumonia.
- It could be related to medications you are taking for high blood pressure, particularly ACE inhibitors. As many as 1 in 5 people develop chronic dry cough as a side effect of their medications. Talk to your doctor to see if another medication might work better for you.

It should now be pretty obvious to you that a simple cough is not always so simple. In the next section, you are going to learn about the various causes of chronic cough in detail – you'll then learn about some of the common symptoms and treatment options for chronic cough.

2. Causes of Chronic Cough

As you learned in the previous section, the three most common causes for chronic cough are postnasal drip, GERD, and asthma. There are, however, many more potential causes for persistent cough, or chronic cough. Here is a list of causes for chronic cough that was developed by Ashok Mahashur and published in the January-February 2015 issue of *Lung India*, a medical journal dedicated to respiratory diseases:

- Upper airway cough syndrome (postnasal drip)
- Cough-variant asthma
- Gastroesophageal reflux disease
- Chronic bronchitis
- Non-acid reflux
- Laryngopharyngeal reflux
- Obstructive sleep apnea
- Vocal cord dysfunction
- Blood pressure medications

There are also some less common causes of chronic cough which include things like lung cancer, cystic fibrosis, sarcoidosis, bronchiolitis, heart disease, and aspiration. In the following pages, you will receive a detailed overview of each of these potential causes for chronic cough.

Upper Airway Cough Syndrome (Postnasal Drip)

Guidelines established in 2006 by the American College of Chest Physicians (ACCP) suggested using the term "upper airway cough syndrome" (UACS) instead of postnasal drip. This change was made because individuals who experience this type of chronic cough may or may not have postnasal drip – it could be related instead to inflammation or irritation of the upper airway that triggers a cough. The most common symptoms associated with UACS include frequent throat clearing, feeling drainage down the back of the throat, and nasal discharge. Two clinical signs also include mucopurulent secretions in the oropharynx and a cobblestone appearance of the oropharyngeal mucosa. Unfortunately, there is no objective test that can be used for UACS – the diagnosis can sometimes only be confirmed if the patient responds to the use of decongestants and/or antihistamines. If the patient doesn't respond, a CT scan may be indicated to identify the underlying cause.

Cough-Variant Asthma

In cases of cough-variant asthma, a chronic dry cough may be the only symptom, or it might just be the predominant one. For most patients with this condition, the cough worsens at night. There are two pathophysiological explanations for the kind of dry cough that is associated with asthma. For one thing, the cough receptors are sensitized by an increase in inflammatory mediators – this leads to an increased cough reflex. Second, the smooth bronchial muscles become constricted which further stimulates the cough receptors. The most reliable test used for diagnosing asthma is called spirometry. If asthma cannot be diagnosed through objective tests, a trial of inhaled corticosteroids can either confirm or rule out the diagnosis, depending on the patient's response. Additional treatments may include bronchodilators, low-dose theophylline, and antileukotrienes.

Gastroesophageal Reflux Disease

As you learned earlier, GERD is the cause for chronic cough in more than 40% of cases. When chronic cough accompanies gastrointestinal symptoms such as heartburn and regurgitation, the first cause to consider is GERD. However, about 75% of patients with GERD do NOT present gastrointestinal symptoms. For this reason, GERD can sometimes be difficult to diagnose. There are three major mechanisms in the body which are associated with GERD-related chronic cough: intraesophageal reflux, laryngopharyngeal reflux, and microaspiration. These three mechanisms either trigger coughing directly or they sensitize the cough reflex, thereby indirectly triggering a cough. Treatment for GERD usually involves lifestyle changes including an anti-reflux diet and acid suppression.

Non-Acid Reflux

As is true with GERD, acid reflux is commonly associated with chronic cough, but it is also possible for non-acid reflux to be involved. Recent studies showed that a small subgroup of patients with chronic cough did not respond to acid suppression treatment but they did improve with antireflux surgery. This suggests that some non-acid gastric components were involved. Similar to acid reflux, non-acid reflux can contribute to a hypersensitive cough reflex by causing inflammation in the airway. The most effective treatments for non-acid reflux include dietary modifications, antireflux surgery, and in some patients, prokinetic drug therapy. Various pH monitoring tests can be used to detect non-acid reflux problems in patients with chronic cough.

Chronic Bronchitis

This condition is part of the COPD spectrum and it is particularly common in people who smoke and in those with high exposure to secondhand smoke. Chronic bronchitis is characterized by prolonged inflammation of the bronchial tubes (the major airways) along with a productive cough that brings up colored sputum. Other symptoms of chronic bronchitis may include wheezing, shortness of breath, low grade fever, and tightness in the chest. Unfortunately, chronic bronchitis is a condition that never really goes away. It can be managed with healthy lifestyle changes and medication, but it can keep coming back.

Laryngopharyngeal Reflux

Also known as LPR, laryngopharyngeal reflux is a commonly accepted cause of chronic cough by otolaryngologists, but pulmonologists have yet to recognize it as such. One reason may be that laryngopharyngeal reflux does not seem to have any specific pathognomonic symptoms or endoscopic findings associated with it. Diagnosis is usually based on laryngoscopic findings such as thickening of the posterior pharynx, erythema, and edema. These same findings are frequently found in patients who have experienced trauma caused by coughing, however, so it is hard to tell the difference between these two conditions.

Obstructive Sleep Apnea

Obstructive sleep apnea is characterized by periodic pauses in breathing during sleep. Basically, your breathing either becomes very shallow or you stop breathing for periods lasting between several seconds and several minutes, and they may occur 30 or more times per hour. Obstructive sleep apnea occurs when something partially or completely blocks the upper airway during sleep – this causes the chest muscles and diaphragm to work harder to pull air into your lungs. Many people with sleep apnea snore and they frequently wake without feeling rested. Recent studies have shown a correlation between chronic cough and obstructive sleep apnea, though the specific mechanism involved is yet unclear. It could be related to an increase in trans-diaphragmatic pressure or upper airway inflammation related to epithelial injury. One trial involving continuous positive airway pressure (CPAP) therapy showed an improvement in the cough of patients with obstructive sleep apnea.

Vocal Cord Dysfunction

This condition occurs when the vocal cords do not open correctly – it is also called paradoxical vocal fold movement. Vocal cord dysfunction (VCD) is sometimes confused with asthma because it presents similar symptoms which may include difficulty breathing, wheezing, coughing, hoarseness, throat tightness, and voice changes. VCD can be diagnosed using a laryngoscope and through spirometric testing. In short-term cases, CPAP treatment can be helpful but voice therapy and lifestyle changes may be needed in chronic cases. Careful management of VCD is crucial, especially in cases where the patient is misdiagnosed with asthma because this can lead to overtreatment with inhaled corticosteroids.

Blood Pressure Medications

Individuals with hypertension (high blood pressure) or heart failure are sometimes treated with medications that have chronic cough as a potential side effect. Some of the medications most commonly associated with this side effect include ACE inhibitors like enalapril and captopril.

Lung Cancer

Lung cancer is a very serious disease that often presents minor symptoms. What starts as a slight shortness of breath can progress to persistent cough, shortness of breath, wheezing, and even coughing up blood. You may also experience symptoms like loss of appetite, weight loss, extreme fatigue, and recurring infections. There are four stages of lung cancer ranging from non-small cell lung cancer where cancer cells are found in the sputum but no tumor has formed to stage IV non-small cell lung cancer that has metastasized throughout the body, often affecting the liver, bones, and brain. Treatment varies depending on the stage and spread of the cancer.

Cystic Fibrosis

An inherited disorder, cystic fibrosis is a condition that causes damage to the lungs, the digestive system, and other organs. It primarily affects the cells in the body that produce mucus, sweat, and digestive enzymes, causing those secretions to thicken and become sticky. Instead of providing lubrication, those secretions form blockages that can contribute to symptoms like persistent cough, wheezing, shortness of breath, exercise intolerance, digestive problems, and repeated lung infections. Cystic fibrosis has no cure but there are treatments to relieve symptoms such as antibiotics to treat lung infections, anti-inflammatory medications to reduce swelling in the lungs, drugs to thin mucus, and inhaled medications to dilate the airways.

Sarcoidosis

Sarcoidosis is an inflammatory condition with no known cause that affects multiple organs, primarily the lungs and lymph glands. This condition may cause shortness of breath and chronic cough in the early stages and might progress to include fever, night sweats, fatigue, swollen joints, and various problems with organs like the kidneys, liver, and heart. Sarcoidosis sometimes presents a sudden appearance of a skin rash along with inflammation of the eyes. There is no cure for sarcoidosis but it frequently improves over time with no treatment in mild cases. When treatment is required, it usually involves healthy lifestyle changes and drug treatment to manage symptoms.

Bronchiolitis

Bronchiolitis is a type of lung infection that is common in young children and infants. It results in congestion and inflammation of the small airways in the lungs known as the bronchioles. This disease is most commonly caused by a virus and it often occurs during the winter. It starts with mild symptoms similar to the common cold then progresses to severe coughing, wheezing, and even breathing problems. Symptoms can last anywhere from several days to several weeks and can be treated with supportive care. Bronchodilators and oral corticosteroid medications have not been found to be particularly effective.

Heart Disease

Heart disease is also known as cardiovascular disease and there are many different types. One of the most severe kinds is congestive heart failure, or simply heart failure, which occurs when the heart fails to pump enough blood throughout the body. Some symptoms of heart failure include shortness of breath, chronic coughing, wheezing and fatigue. These things happen because, as blood travels from the lungs into the heart, it sometimes backs up into the lungs, making breathing more difficult. Heart failure can also cause fluid retention, rapid heartbeat, and confusion. Treatment for heart failure usually involves relieving symptoms and improving quality of life through lifestyle changes and medication. Surgery may also be used to correct structural problems.

Now that you know more about some of the underlying conditions that can contribute to chronic cough, you may be wondering about what other symptoms you might experience. In the next section, we'll go into detail about common symptoms for chronic cough and then we'll move into diagnosis and treatment options.

3. Symptoms for Chronic Cough

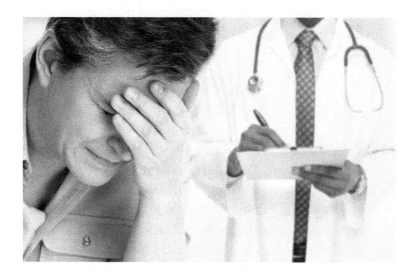

You already know what a cough is, and you've already learned what makes chronic cough different from acute cough. But let's quickly review the symptoms of chronic cough as well as some of the potential complications. A chronic cough can be either productive (producing mucus) or non-productive. <u>Along with the cough itself, you may also experience symptoms such as those listed below</u>:

- Stuffy or runny nose
- Postnasal drip (liquid running down throat)
- Sore or scratchy throat
- Hoarseness or loss of voice
- Frequent clearing your throat
- Wheezing or shortness of breath
- Heartburn or chest pain
- Sour taste in your mouth
- Coughing up blood

Some complications you may experience as a side effect of your chronic cough could include things like headache or dizziness, excessive sweating, loss of bladder control, fractured ribs, extreme fatigue, and even passing out.

4. Diagnosis and Treatment for Persistent Cough

If you experience a cold lasting more than 1 week, you should consider seeing your doctor in order to identify the underlying cause. Even after you seek initial treatment, you should consider going back to your doctor if your cough lasts longer than 3 weeks. In many cases, your primary care physician will be qualified to diagnose chronic cough, though you may want to go to the emergency room if it is severe enough to cause breathing difficulties or other serious symptoms. Your doctor (or the ER specialist) may then refer to you a specialist.

One of the specialists that you might see is called a pulmonologist – this is a doctor who specializes in treating diseases of the lungs and airway. If it is determined that your chronic cough is related to allergies, you may be referred to an allergist. A gastroenterologist is who you should see if your persistent cough is related to GERD and, if it is secondary to heart disease, you will see a cardiologist.

When you go to see the doctor for your chronic cough, they will perform a number of tests and evaluations. First, your doctor will take your medical history and perform a physical exam. At this time, you should tell your doctor about all of your symptoms, when they started, and how they have progressed. Depending on the information you give them, your doctor may then order tests to identify the underlying cause of the issue. These tests may include blood tests, sputum tests, and lab sample tests. If your doctor wants to check for lung cancer or pneumonia, they might order a chest X-ray or a CT scan.

Once your doctor has identified the cause of your chronic cough, they will recommend a course of treatment. Again, the recommended course of treatment will vary depending on the cause of your persistent cough, especially if there is more than one underlying condition. If your problem is caused by allergies or a sinus infection, you may be prescribed some kind of glucocorticoid, decongestant, or antihistamine. For asthma problems, an inhaled corticosteroid or bronchodilator may help. Antibiotics can be used to treat bacterial infections that cause chronic cough and acid blockers may be helpful in cases of GERD. If the cause can't be determined, your doctor may just treat the cough itself with cough suppressants.

Now that you know a little more about chronic cough (or persistent cough), including its symptoms and causes, you can see how it differs from other kinds of coughs. In the next chapter, we are going to discuss dry cough in greater detail, including interesting facts and statistics, symptoms, and potential causes.

Chapter 3: Causes of Dry Cough

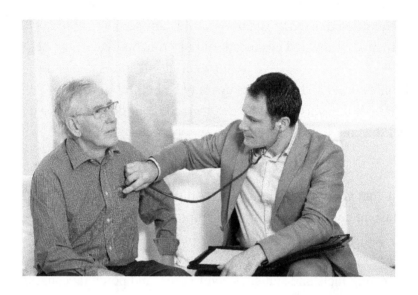

You've already learned that coughs are generally divided into two categories – productive and unproductive. But another way to think of them is as wet coughs versus dry coughs. Wet coughs are so named because they bring up sputum but a dry cough is nonproductive, so it doesn't. When you have a dry cough, you might feel a lump or tickle in your throat but no amount of coughing will make it go away.

In this chapter, you are going to learn all you have ever wanted to know about dry cough. We'll start with some interesting facts and statistics about dry cough then move on to the potential causes for this kind of cough. We'll finish up with detailed information about the symptoms and treatment options for dry cough.

1. Facts and Statistics

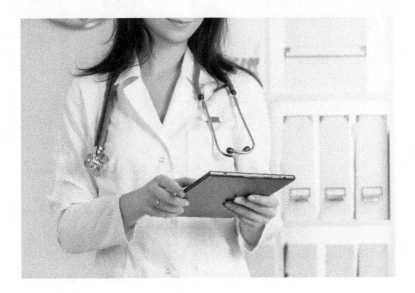

A dry cough can become persistent if it lasts for more than a few weeks and many of the causes for dry cough overlap with those of chronic cough. Some of the most common causes for dry cough include allergies, asthma, COPD and GERD, though there are also some less common causes you should be aware of. Before we get into the details, however, let's take a look at some interesting facts and statistics about various types of dry cough. <u>Below you will find some facts and statistics about different types of dry cough</u>:

- In 2014, the CDC identified a 15% increase in the number of reported cases for pertussis, or whooping cough.
- There are about 16 million cases of pertussis worldwide each year and it is responsible for nearly 200,000 deaths.
- Cases of whooping cough can last for 10 weeks or longer, giving this disease the nickname the "100-day cough".

- Each year, approximately 5% to 20% of the American population will get the flu and 200,000 people will be hospitalized for it.
- It usually takes 1 to 4 days for flu symptoms to develop but you can be contagious from the first day until 5 to 10 days after symptoms appear.
- The average cost for treatment of flu, including hospitalizations and outpatient treatment, is over $10 billion.
- To date, six times as many women as men have died of COPD – this continues to be the same today.
- COPD affects about 12 million adults in the United States each year and as many as 120,000 die from it annually.
- It is estimated that as many as 10% to 20% of COPD patients have never smoked a cigarette, which suggests that there is an involvement of genetic and environmental factors in developing the disease.
- Pneumonia accounts for more than 15% of deaths in children under the age of 5 – it killed more than 900,000 children worldwide in 2015.
- Though pneumonia is less often fatal for children in the United States than in other countries, it is still the #1 reason for hospitalization of children in the U.S.
- The overuse of antibiotics, both in and outside the hospital, has led to a growth in antibiotic resistance in the bacteria known to cause pneumonia.
- Even after successful treatment, pneumonia can lead to long-term consequences like cardiovascular disease, cognitive decline, and increased risk of lung diseases.
- Mental factors such as chronic stress can produce a psychogenic cough that increases in periods of stress and goes away during sleep.

If you ask a doctor, you will find that there are actually three different kinds of dry cough. The first is a dry hacking cough, the kind that is usually associated with infections of the nose and throat. With this cough, you may feel like you have something stuck in your throat but coughing will not make it go away. The second type is a barking cough, also known as croup. This type of cough is usually associated with laryngitis and it may cause both pain and difficulty breathing. The third type of whooping cough, also known as pertussis, is caused by bacteria.

In some cases, dry cough is a lingering symptom from some kind of infection or other disease. The longer the dry cough lasts, the more irritated and inflamed your throat can become. Though you should talk to your doctor about treatment for the underlying cause of your dry cough, there are certain natural remedies which may help to soothe your sore throat and reduce your cough. Here are some natural remedies for dry cough:

- Gargling saltwater
- Drinking warm liquid
- Using Vapo-rub
- Sucking on throat lozenges
- Sleeping with head elevated
- Herbal tea with honey

Once you have experienced dry cough – particularly chronic dry cough – you will not be eager to experience it again. Fortunately, there are some simple things you can do to help prevent this cough in the future. Here are some things to try:

- Wash your hands with hot water and soap
- Cover your mouth when sneezing or coughing
- Avoid eating too close to bedtime
- Don't sleep flat on your back

- Do not smoke
- Moderate consumption of caffeinated beverages
- Don't overexert yourself
- Do not eat too many cold foods

In the next section, you are going to learn about the various causes that can be associated with dry cough. You'll then learn about some of the common symptoms as well as diagnosis methods and treatment options for dry cough.

2. Causes of Dry Cough

As was mentioned earlier, some of the most common causes of dry cough include allergies, asthma, GERD, and COPD. There are, however, many conditions that may include dry cough as a symptom. <u>Here is a list of some of the potential causes of dry cough, including some that are fairly uncommon:</u>

- Allergies
- Asthma
- Cold or flu
- COPD
- GERD
- HIV
- Inhaled irritants
- Laryngitis
- Pneumonia
- Psychogenic cough
- Stress
- Tuberculosis
- Whooping cough

In the following pages, you will receive a detailed overview of each of these potential causes for dry cough.

Allergies and Asthma

In many cases, patients who suffer from asthma experience symptoms of breathlessness and wheezing, but there are also some who only experience a dry cough. Asthma is caused by bronchospasm which can be triggered by exposure to certain allergens like dust or mold as well as cold air or exercise. In asthma patients who experience dry cough, it can happen around the clock but often starts at night. Treatment options for cough-variant asthma include bronchodilator sprays like albuterol and inhaled corticosteroids like triamcinolone and fluticasone.

Cold or Flu

At this point in your life, you have undoubtedly had a cold or two and you may have also had the flu at some point in time. Both of these conditions can cause coughs and they often present with similar symptoms. A cold usually begins with a sore throat which can progress to nasal symptoms, congestion, and cough. The symptoms of a cold usually improve within a week. If they don't, it may be a bacterial infection. Flu symptoms are similar to cold symptoms but they are more severe and tend to come on more quickly. You may have a sore throat, headache, fever, muscle aches, congestion, and cough.

COPD

Short for chronic obstructive pulmonary disease, COPD is a progressive disease that frequently causes coughing. Technically, COPD is a group of diseases that includes bronchitis and emphysema, so smoking is the leading cause of this condition. You can also get COPD from prolonged exposure to secondhand smoke or other irritants like chemical fumes, dust, and air pollution. COPD is the third leading cause of death in the United

States, so it is very serious. Symptoms tend to develop slowly and worsen over time. For many people, it starts with a dry cough that tends to linger and does not improve when treated with over-the-counter cough remedies. There is currently no cure for COPD, though surgical treatments and medications can be used to improve and manage the symptoms.

GERD

Though many GERD patients experience heartburn as their main symptom, some complain more of a chronic dry cough. GERD is a disease that occurs when stomach acid backs up into the esophagus, causing irritation of the lower esophagus which can stimulate the cough reflex and cause a sore throat to develop. Many patients who have GERD experience recurrent bouts of laryngitis and an unexplained sore throat as well.

HIV

HIV is a type of virus that attacks the immune system, targeting white blood cells called T cells. As the virus grows stronger, the immune system grows weaker and the body becomes unable to protect itself against infection. Without treatment, HIV can progress to AIDS which is usually fatal. A dry cough is a common symptom for HIV but, on its own, it is not enough to indicate this condition. When accompanied by flu-like symptoms, swelling of the lymph nodes, nausea, and rash, it could be HIV.

Inhaled Irritants

Whether or not you have allergies or asthma, inhaling various environmental irritants can trigger your cough reflex. This is particularly common with allergens like mold, dust, and dander but can also happen with workplace chemicals like sulfur dioxide and nitric oxide. In some cases, even clean air can trigger your cough reflex if it is very cold or if you have been exercising vigorously.

Laryngitis

Laryngitis is a type of inflammation of the larynx (voice box) typically due to infection, irritation, or overuse. In a healthy individual, the vocal cords open and close smoothly to create speech but in cases of laryngitis, they become irritated or inflamed which can cause distortion of speech akin to hoarseness. Laryngitis can be either acute or chronic and it may be accompanied or preceded by a dry cough. Cases of acute laryngitis typically resolve on their own but if it lasts more than 3 weeks you should seek medical attention because the symptoms may be caused by exposure to chemical irritants.

Pneumonia

Pneumonia is a lung infection caused by bacteria or viruses and it can cause fever, breathing difficulty, and coughing. In many cases, pneumonia causes a wet cough that produces sputum, but sometimes people who recover from pneumonia experience a lingering dry cough related to irritation and inflammation in the lungs and throat. Pneumonia can also increase a person's risk of developing other lung diseases down the road.

Psychogenic Cough

Also known as habit cough, psychogenic cough is generally not associated with any biological illness or physical stimulus, though it may start out that way. Psychogenic cough usually produces a harsh, tinny sound and it can persist for weeks or even months with coughs occurring as frequently as every 2 to 3 seconds. This kind of cough can be diagnosed when no obvious organic basis can be identified – it also tends to disappear completely when the individual is asleep. Conventional cough medicine will have no effect but speech therapy, suggestion therapy, and self-hypnosis techniques may be effective.

Stress

You may already be familiar with the negative effects of stress on the body, but did you know that it can also cause cough? Cough caused by stress is sometimes called anxiety cough because it tends to manifest during periods of extreme stress or anxiety. Because this type of cough is triggered by anxiety and stress, it will come and go and vary in intensity. This kind of cough tends to diminish at night and during periods of rest, though for some it can worsen throughout the day and escalate at night.

Tuberculosis

Though once incredibly deadly and highly contagious, tuberculosis is now under some degree of control and there is a vaccine available. Tuberculosis is a bacterial infection that causes flu-like symptoms including fever, chills, night sweats, and loss of appetite – it also causes coughs. The bacteria responsible for this disease typically affect the lungs but can spread to other organs including the liver, kidneys, heart, and brain. Tuberculosis can be cured with antibiotic treatment.

Whooping Cough

Also known as pertussis, whooping cough is a type of respiratory tract infection. This condition gets its name because following each dry cough comes a gasping of air that makes a "whooping" sound. Whooping cough can last for several weeks and individual coughing spells can last for a minute or longer. This condition is particularly dangerous for children under the age of 6, largely because they are too young to receive the vaccine. Antibiotics can be used to kill the bacteria responsible for the disease but you should avoid over-the-counter cough remedies because they won't work and they may interact with the antibiotics.

Now that we've covered some of the underlying conditions that can cause dry cough, you may be wondering about what other symptoms you might experience. In the next section, we'll go into detail about common symptoms for dry cough and then we'll finish up with an overview of diagnosis and treatment options.

3. Symptoms for Dry Cough

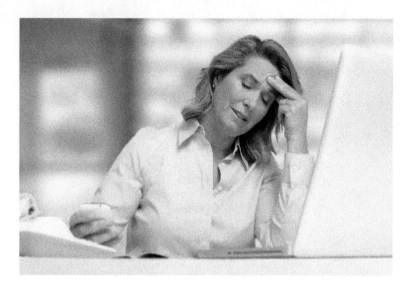

You've probably experienced a dry cough at some point during your life, so you may already know what it feels like. Dry cough can be scratchy or even painful, causing your throat to become increasingly more irritated the longer it lasts. <u>Along with the cough itself, you may also experience symptoms such as those listed below</u>:

- Persistent tickle in the throat
- Feeling a lump in the throat
- Dryness or sore throat
- No wheezing or congestion
- Coughing worsens at night

Depending on how severe your dry cough is and how long it lasts, you may also experience some unpleasant side effects or complications. For example, the cough could impact your ability to breathe which could cause you to faint. Sometimes severe coughing fits can lead to fractured ribs, vomiting, or muscle pain. Seek medical attention for a cough lasting longer than 7 days.

4. Diagnosis and Treatment for Dry Cough

If you are worried that your dry cough is caused by an underlying condition, or if it lasts for more than 7 days, you should see your doctor. When you go to see the doctor, they will perform a number of tests and evaluations. First, they will complete a medical history and perform a physical exam. During the exam, be sure to tell your doctor about all of your symptoms, when they started, and how they have progressed over time. Depending on the information you give them, your doctor may then order tests to identify the underlying cause of the dry cough. If your doctor wants to check for pneumonia or other infections, they might order a chest x-ray or a CT scan.

Once your doctor has identified the cause of your dry cough, they will recommend a course of treatment. As you already know, the recommended course of treatment will vary depending on the cause of your dry cough. If your problem is caused by allergies or asthma, you may be prescribed some kind of glucocorticoid, or antihistamine. For viral infections like cold and flu, you may just need to stay hydrated and use cough drops and hot liquids to soothe your sore throat. Antibiotics can be used to treat bacterial infections and acid blockers may be helpful in cases of GERD. If the cause for your dry cough can't be determined, your doctor may just treat the cough naturally.

At this point you should have a thorough understanding of dry cough, including its symptoms and causes. You can now see how it differs from chronic cough, or persistent cough. In the next chapter, we are going to discuss the stages of persistent cough. You'll learn how to identify the type of cough you have and learn about the signs of onset.

Chapter 4: The Stages of a Cough

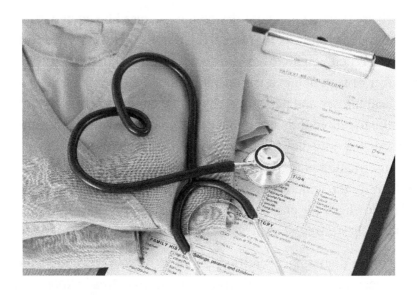

Many people use the words "cold" and "cough" interchangeably, though a cold is technically a disease and a cough is a symptom. You've probably had more than a few colds throughout the course of your life, but have you ever taken the time to really break things down and think about how it works? In this chapter, we are going to review the stages of a cough (or cold) but first we'll talk about what a cough is. You'll learn about your cough reflex and exactly what happens in your body when you cough.

Once you understand the mechanism of a cough, we're going to review different types of coughs. The type of cough you have will help you to determine the underlying cause. You've already learned the differences between dry cough and wet cough, acute cough and chronic cough, but I'll give you some simple questions to answer so you can narrow down the cause of your cough.

Finally, we'll talk about the stages of the common cold so you can see how a simple cough might turn into something else.

1. What is a Cough?

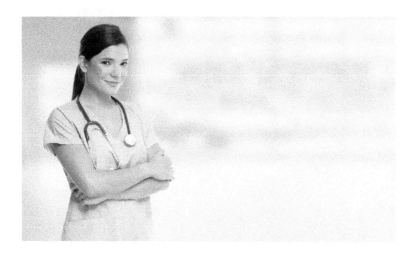

At this point you have learned all about the different kinds of coughs and their relevant causes, but what exactly is a cough? A cough is a protective reflex that the body employs to clear debris or excessive secretions from the airway. In many cases, you cough when your cough reflex is triggered – there are three components to the cough reflex:

- Afferent sensory limb
- Central processing center
- Efferent limb

Throughout your airway, there are a variety of different receptors but there are three main types. Rapidly adapting receptors (RARs) respond to mechanical stimuli (like something tickling your throat) as well as things like cigarette smoke, chemical fumes, and pulmonary congestion. You also have slowly adapting receptors (SARs) and nociceptors which respond to chemical stimuli and inflammatory or immunological mediators.

When the afferent sensory limb receives an impulse, it transmits that impulse to the central processing center – the cough center in your brain. This is connected to the central respiratory generator which controls your breathing. The impulse then travels to the larynx and sends signals to the intercostal muscles as well as the muscles in your abdominal wall, your diaphragm, and your pelvic floor. These are all of the muscles that become involved when you cough – try coughing now to see if you can feel them.

2. What Kind of Cough Do You Have?

If you go to the doctor for a cough or cold, they will ask you some questions about your symptoms. These questions are used to identify your symptoms more clearly and to work towards a diagnosis. <u>If you want to get an idea what the underlying cause for your cough might be, ask yourself these questions</u>:

Do you have a heavy cough with lots of mucus?

When you have a heavy, mucus cough you may feel as though there is a heavy weight resting on your chest. You may also have a strong cough that produces a lot of mucus. This type of cough occurs when your body begins to produce excess mucus in order to trap bacteria, viruses, or other pathogens to help expel them from the body by coughing.

Do you have a chesty cough with congestion?

When you have a chesty cough, it might feel like someone is squeezing your chest, causing it to feel tight. This type of cough is caused by an accumulation of mucus or phlegm around the lungs – this is known as chest congestion. This is a common symptom of respiratory tract infections.

Do you have a tickling cough in your throat?

When you have a tickling cough, it can be very irritating, both physically and mentally. It might feel like someone is tickling your throat with a feather and no amount of coughing seems to relieve the sensation. This kind of cough is usually the result of throat irritation and it often results in a sore throat.

Do you have a long-lasting dry cough?

When you have a dry cough, it may feel like there is a lump in your throat but coughing doesn't produce anything. After a time, a persistent dry cough can become very intense and sometimes painful and you tend to feel it more in your throat than in your chest. This kind of cough is usually caused by irritation in the upper airway and is sometimes secondary to an infection like the cold or flu. It may also be triggered by environmental irritants such as cigarette smoke, dust, and fumes.

3. The Progression of a Cough

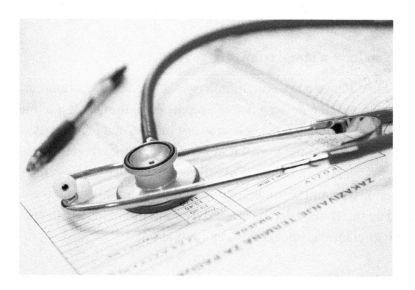

The life cycle of the common cold usually lasts between 7 and 10 days, though you may not develop symptoms immediately after exposure. Though colds are very common, they can be caused by hundreds of different viruses – this makes it difficult to identify the specific pathogen and also makes some treatment ineffective. Here is how a cold typically progresses:

Exposure – You can be exposed to the cold virus by making direct contact with someone who is infected or by breathing the same air.

Day 1 and 2 – About one to two days after exposure, you may start to develop cold symptoms. At first you might feel a tickle in your throat and you may start sneezing more than usual. When you feel a cold coming on, it is important to drink plenty of fluids and to get lots of rest.

Day 3 to 5 – After about three days, you'll start to experience nasal symptoms like runny nose and congestion. As day three turns to day four, your nasal discharge may become thicker and develop a yellow or greenish tint. By day five, postnasal drip and sore throat may cause you to develop a cough.

Days 6 and 7 – Once you've gotten through the first five days, your symptoms should start to ease and you'll begin to feel a little bit better. If you haven't improved or if your symptoms get worse after this point, talk to your doctor.

Days 8 to 10 – By this time, most of your symptoms should have gone away. You may have a lingering cough if your throat was particularly irritated, but your congestion and nasal discharge should be gone and you'll start getting your energy back as well.

Chapter 5: Chronic, Dry Cough Treatment

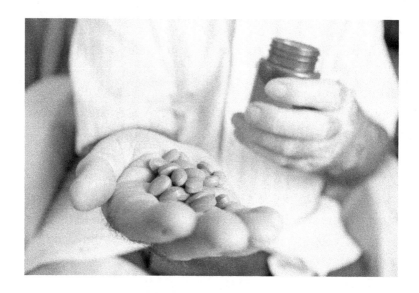

When you have a cough, you want to make it go away as soon as possible. Unfortunately, if you have chronic cough things may not be as easy as you would like. Finding the right treatment that will kick your cough to the curb can be tricky because there are so many potential underlying causes. If you want to relieve your cough quickly, you might consider some over-the-counter cough remedies like cough syrup or cough drops. If you don't like taking medication, there are plenty of natural remedies you can try. You'll learn about both of these as well as some methods for preventing cough in this chapter.

1. Medical Treatment Options

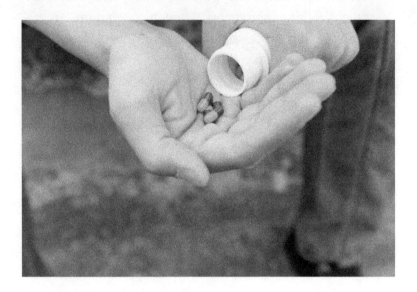

If you walk into your local drug store you will find at least one aisle filled with different cough treatments. You'll find everything from syrups and sprays to tablets, lozenges, and more. In fact, it is estimated that Americans spend as much as $3.5 billion each year on prescription and over-the-counter cough remedies. <u>Here is an overview of some of the most common cough remedies and how they work</u>:

- **Antihistamines** – These over-the-counter remedies are the most effective in treating cough related to allergies and postnasal drip. These medications work by drying out secretions which can be a good thing for some coughs, but may also make sputum harder to expel. Antihistamines also frequently cause sleepiness.
- **Cough Drops** – Sucking on a cough drop can help to moisturize a dry throat and, depending on the ingredients

used, may have an analgesic effect. Many cough drops contain menthol, eucalyptus oil, honey, camphor, and other soothing ingredients. Though cough drops are immensely popular, there is no definitive evidence to suggest that they are more effective in relieving a cough than regular hard candies.

- **Cough Suppressant**s – These remedies work by suppressing the cough reflex. This can be beneficial in cases of dry cough but with wet cough you want to cough to remove sputum. There are over-the-counter remedies made with dextromethorphan which work fairly well, though codeine is more effective.
- **Decongestants** – Many cough remedies contain decongestants but they really only work for cough caused by sinusitis or postnasal drip. Decongestant medications also frequently contain topical anesthetics like benzocaine to help desensitize the nerves responsible for triggering the cough reflex.
- **Expectorants** – This type of medication is designed to help loosen sputum so that it is easier to clear – one of the most popular expectorants is called guaifenesin. According to numerous studies, expectorants are no more or less effective than drinking lots of water and using a humidifier.
- **Lozenges** – Similar to cough drops, lozenges may contain camphor, menthol, honey, and other substances known to help relieve cough.

Because cough remedies come in a variety of different forms (many of which offer a combination of therapies), you need to be very careful about which one you choose. Your best bet is to speak to the in-store pharmacist and describe your symptoms so that they can direct you to the proper treatment. No matter which remedy you choose, be sure to follow dosing instructions very carefully. Keep in mind that some treatments will interact poorly with alcohol or other medications you may be taking.

2. Tips for Prevention

There is no fireproof way to prevent a cough – it is up to your immune system to fight off the bacteria, virus, or other pathogen causing it. But there are certain things you can do in your daily life to help protect you against sickness. Here are some of the top things to do to prevent dry cough and chronic cough:

- Wash your hands frequently – especially during cold and flu season – using hot water and soap for 20 to 30 seconds.
- Avoid contact with people who are sick – consider wearing a mask or gloves when you can't prevent exposure.
- Do not smoke or use any other forms of tobacco and try to avoid exposure to secondhand smoke.
- Keep your body hydrated by drinking plenty of fluids – this will help to keep your mucus thin.
- Get a flu shot every year to protect yourself against influenza.
- If you are 65 or older, get a pneumococcal vaccine to protect yourself against pneumonia – especially if you have COPD, asthma, chronic lung disease, or are a smoker.
- Stay up to date on your immunizations, especially for whooping cough (pertussis).
- Eat and drink plenty of foods that are rich in vitamin C and other immune-boosting nutrients.

In addition to doing these simple things to avoid getting sick yourself, you should also take precautions against getting other people sick. If you use communal facilities like a gym or a computer lab, be sure to wash your hands before touching equipment and wipe the equipment clean after you are done. If you are sick, always cover your coughing and sneezing, but not with your hands – sneeze or cough into your elbow.

3. Natural and Herbal Remedies

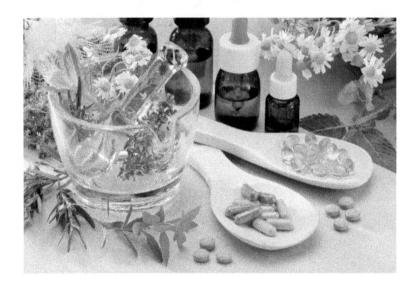

If you don't like the idea of putting chemicals into your body, you will be glad to know that there are many natural and herbal remedies out there for coughs. There are some simple things you can do such as taking a hot shower, drinking tea, or gargling saltwater. You can also use things like honey, fresh herbs and spices, and essential oils to make your own natural cough remedies at home. In the following pages, you will receive a collection of homemade cough remedies including cough syrups, cough drops, tonics, steam inhalations, and more.

a. Homemade Remedies for Cough

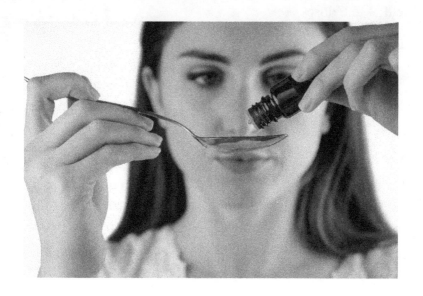

<u>Recipes Included in this Section</u>:

Honey Lemon Cough Syrup

Ginger Peppermint Cough Syrup

Lemon Bourbon Cough Reliever

Cayenne Cough Syrup

Herbal Throat Spray

Honey Cinnamon Cough Drops

Ginger Clove Cough Drops

Herbed Menthol Cough Drops

Eucalyptus Steam Inhalation

Slippery Elm Throat Lozenges

Honey Lemon Cough Syrup

Yield: 4 to 6 doses

Ingredients:

- 1 tablespoon coconut oil
- 2 tablespoons honey
- 1 to 2 tablespoons fresh lemon juice

Instructions:

1. Melt the coconut oil in a small saucepan over low heat.
2. Remove from heat, whisk in the honey and lemon juice.
3. Take by the spoonful as needed or stir into hot water or tea and sip slowly.

Ginger Peppermint Cough Syrup

Yield: about 1 ½ cups

Ingredients:

- 1 ½ tablespoons fresh grated ginger
- 1 ½ teaspoons dried peppermint
- 2 cups water
- ½ cup honey

Instructions:

1. Combine the ginger and peppermint in a saucepan.
2. Pour in the water then bring to a boil.
3. Reduce heat and simmer on low until reduced by half.
4. Strain the liquid into a glass jar and stir in the honey until it is completely dissolved.
5. Take 1 tablespoon every 3 to 4 hours to ease the cough.

6. Keep the extra refrigerated up to 3 weeks.

Cayenne Cough Syrup

Yield: 8 to 10 doses

Ingredients:

- ¼ cup water
- 2 tablespoons honey
- 2 tablespoons apple cider vinegar
- ½ teaspoon ground ginger
- ¼ to ½ teaspoon cayenne

Instructions:

1. Warm the water in a small saucepan over low heat.
2. When the water is hot, stir in the honey until it melts.
3. Remove from heat and stir in the apple cider vinegar, ginger, and cayenne.
4. Take one teaspoon as needed to relieve cough.

Lemon Bourbon Cough Reliever

Yield: 1 dose

Ingredients:

- 2 tablespoons bourbon
- 2 tablespoons fresh lemon juice
- ¼ cup water
- Honey to taste

Instructions:

1. Whisk together the bourbon, lemon juice, and water in a microwave safe container.
2. Heat the mixture for about 45 seconds until steaming.
3. Stir in the honey then heat for another 30 to 45 seconds.
4. Let the syrup cool a little bit then sip slowly.

Herbal Throat Spray

Ingredients:

- 2 teaspoons dried ginger
- 2 teaspoons dried Echinacea
- 2 teaspoons dried elderberry
- 2 teaspoons dried thyme
- 2 teaspoons dried marshmallow root
- 2 tablespoons boiling water
- 40-proof vodka or rum, as needed
- 1 tablespoon honey

Instructions:

1. Combine the dried herbs in a glass half-pint jar.
2. Pour in the boiling water then fill the jar the rest of the way with high-quality vodka or rum (at least 40-proof).
3. Seal the jar with the lid and let rest in a cool, dark place for at least 2 weeks.
4. Combine three tablespoons of the herb tincture with the honey in a small spray bottle.
5. Use the throat spray to relieve the sore throat and cough.

Honey Cinnamon Cough Drops

Ingredients:

- ½ cup cold-pressed coconut oil
- ½ cup honey
- 1 teaspoon ground Ceylon cinnamon

Instructions:

1. Spoon the coconut oil into a mixing bowl and beat with an electric mixer until whipped.
2. Beat in the honey and cinnamon until well combined.
3. Pour the mixture into small silicone molds and freeze until solid, about 15 to 20 minutes.
4. Pop the cough drops out of the mold and store in an airtight container in the refrigerator.

Ginger Clove Cough Drops

Ingredients:

- ½ cup water
- 1 cup white sugar
- 1 tablespoon honey
- 2 to 3 teaspoons fresh lemon juice
- ½ teaspoon ground ginger
- ¼ teaspoon ground cloves
- Powdered sugar or cornstarch, as needed

Instructions:

1. Line a baking sheet with parchment then grease with cooking spray and set aside.
2. Whisk together the water, sugar, honey, lemon juice, ginger, and cloves in a small saucepan.
3. Cook the mixture on medium heat, stirring often, until it reaches 300°F on a candy thermometer.

4. You can test the mixture by dropping a little into a bowl of ice water – if it cracks it is ready.
5. Remove saucepan from heat and let mixture cool a little.
6. Drop the mixture in teaspoon-sized rounds on the prepared baking sheet.
7. Let the drops cool completely then dust with powdered sugar or cornstarch to keep them separated.
8. Store in an airtight container in a cool, dry location.

Eucalyptus Steam Inhalation

Ingredients:

- 4 cups water
- 2 to 3 drops eucalyptus essential oil

Instructions:

1. Bring the water to boil in a saucepan over medium-high heat.
2. Pour the water into a heatproof bowl then place it on a trivet on the table in front of you.
3. Add the eucalyptus oil then drape a towel over your head and lean over the bowl.
4. Breathe gently for 10 to 15 minutes to clear congestion.

Slippery Elm Throat Lozenges

Ingredients:

- ¼ cup boiling water
- 2 tablespoons honey
- ¼ cup slippery elm powder

Instructions:

1. Combine the boiling water and honey in a heatproof bowl.
2. Stir until the honey dissolves.
3. Place the slippery elm powder in a separate bowl then pour the warmed mixture over it.
4. Mix the ingredients well then roll into small balls by hand.
5. To keep the balls from sticking together, roll them in a little extra slippery elm powder.
6. Spread the balls on a parchment-lined baking sheet and let them dry out before using.

Herbed Menthol Cough Drops

Ingredients:

- Coconut oil, as needed
- 3 bags "throat coat" tea
- 1 ¼ cups water
- 1 cup honey
- ¼ teaspoon menthol crystals
- 15 drops peppermint essential oil
- 12 drops lemon essential oil
- 12 drops eucalyptus essential oil
- 6 drops lavender essential oil
- 6 drops tea tree essential oil
- Powdered sugar, optional

Instructions:

1. Grease a set of small candy molds with coconut oil then set them aside.
2. Place the tea bags and water in a small saucepan and bring to a boil.

3. Reduce heat and simmer for 5 minutes then remove from heat and cover.
4. Let the tea bags steep for 15 minutes then squeeze them to release as much liquid as possible.
5. Place the saucepan over medium heat then stir in honey.
6. Bring the mixture to a boil then reduce heat and simmer until the mixture reaches 300°F.
7. Remove from heat then stir in the menthol crystals along with the essentials oils.
8. Stir well then pour into the candy molds and let harden.
9. Pop the cough drops out of the molds and wrap individually or dust with powdered sugar to keep them from sticking together.

Chapter 6: Diet Tips for Persistent Cough

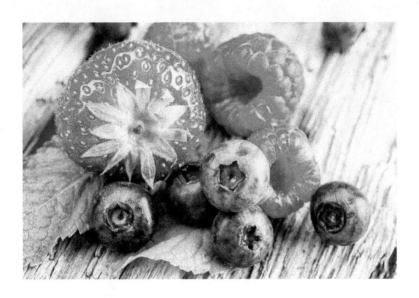

You've probably heard the saying, "You are what you eat." While you probably won't turn into a quarter pounder with cheese, you should know that the things you eat have a direct impact on your health and wellness. The human body is like a machine – when it is properly maintained and gets the right kind of energy, it runs like clockwork. But when you let the machine fall into disrepair, all of the parts slowly stop working as they should and eventually the whole thing will fail.

While it is easy to understand how a healthy diet can improve your overall health and wellbeing, we often don't think about specific foods that can help with specific problems. For example, there are many foods that can help you to recover more quickly from your chronic cough – there are also some foods that could make it worse. In this chapter, you'll receive a detailed list of foods that are bad for coughs and those that are good for coughs.

You'll also receive a collection of delicious cough-busting recipes for natural cough cures and tasty meals and snacks.

1. What Foods are Bad for Coughs?

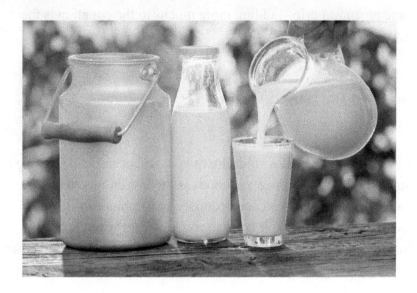

You have already learned the difference between acute cough and chronic cough, as well as the difference between productive and unproductive cough. Whether triggered by allergies, asthma, excess mucus, or whatever else, a cough is a bodily reflex designed to clear the airway. Certain foods you eat may cause your body to produce more mucus or thicker mucus, and there are some foods that can trigger asthma attacks or GERD. In the following pages, you will receive an overview of some of the top foods that are bad for coughs.

Milk and Dairy

Milk and other dairy products contain a protein that stimulates mucus production during digestion. As your intestinal tract begins to produce more mucus, your respiratory tract might jump on the train as well. If you already have a cough, you probably also have some postnasal drip – adding more mucus to the equation is the last thing you need.

Processed Foods

If you are fighting off a cold, flu, or some other infection, eating a bunch of unhealthy processed foods is the last thing you need. Poor nutrition habits can compromise your immune system, making it harder for your body to recover from your cough. Rather than reaching for packaged snacks, baked goods, and other processed foods, stick to whole foods that are nutrient-dense.

Fried Foods

Fried foods are bad for a cough in the same way that processed foods are, but they are also bad in a different way. The process of frying foods releases into the air an irritant called acrolein. Airborne irritants like this can trigger coughing episodes, particularly in people with asthma and those who are already suffering from chronic cough.

Mango, Banana, and Citrus

Though mangoes, bananas, and citrus fruits are all full of nutrients, you may want to avoid these foods if you already have a cough. These foods have high acid content which can contribute to reflux. If you already have GERD, you want to avoid acidic foods like the plague. But if you just have a cough, the acid in these foods can cause further irritation and may also cause acid reflux that can trigger your cough reflex. Instead, focus on fruits with high water content like melons, peaches, and pears.

Caffeinated Beverages

When you are suffering from chronic cough, particularly if it is the result of a cold or flu, staying hydrated is of the utmost importance. While water, tea, and fruit juices can help you stay hydrated, caffeinated beverages can have the opposite effect. In addition to giving you a boost of energy, caffeine also boosts your urination – it acts as a diuretic that flushes fluids from your body more quickly than usual. Dehydration can lead to that dry, scratchy cough that irritates your throat.

Alcoholic Beverages

Alcoholic beverages have a similar effect on your immune system to processed foods. Though the immune-suppressing effects of alcohol may be short-lived, you really want to avoid anything that can make your cough last longer. It is also important to note that alcohol can interact with some over-the-counter cold remedies, especially those that contain sedatives.

2. What Foods are Good for Coughs?

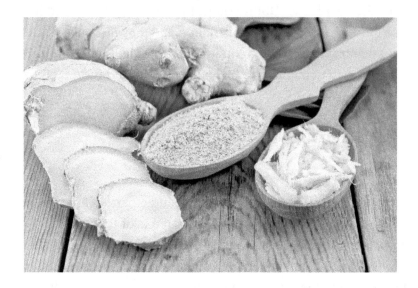

The best thing you can do for your body when you have a cough is to fuel up with healthy, nutritious foods. In general, you should be shying away from processed foods and convenience foods, focusing instead on wholesome, natural foods like lean protein, healthy fats, fresh fruits and vegetables, and natural herbs and spices. In the following pages, you will receive an overview of some of the specific foods that are good for helping your body to recover more quickly from persistent cough.

Here are some natural herbs and spices that will boost your immunity and relieve your cough:

- **Anise** – This spice is probably not one that you use very often but it is very effective for bronchial ailments as well as chest congestion and cough because it is a natural expectorant. It is best used in tea form.

- **Cardamom** – Like anise, cardamom is a natural expectorant – it also has natural antioxidant content. Cardamom helps to improve blood pressure and can help to detoxify caffeine from your system as well.
- **Cinnamon** – This flavorful spice has natural warming properties and it is also great for your immune system as an anti-inflammatory, antibacterial, and antioxidant spice. It is particularly powerful when combined with honey.
- **Garlic** – Not only is garlic loaded with flavor, but it has natural antibacterial and antiviral properties that can boost your immunity as well. Garlic contains allicin and other compounds that can help to fortify your immune system.
- **Ginger** – This root has a natural hotness to it that will help to clear up your congestion. Ginger tea sweetened with honey is great for loosening mucus.
- **Honey** – Though technically not an herb or spice, honey is a common ingredient in herbal remedies for cold and cough. It soothes sore throats that are raw from persistent cough and can be used to sweeten herbal tea.
- **Peppermint** – Most of the benefits associated with the peppermint herb are digestive which can be good for people suffering from GERD. Peppermint tea is also a good remedy for mild cough.
- **Rosemary** – This fragrant herb acts as a natural digestive aid and it has been shown to stimulate the immune system as well. Rosemary is also loaded with antioxidants and, when used in tea, can relieve asthma and cough symptoms.
- **Thyme** – This herb has powerful antimicrobial properties and it can also help to fight against bacteria and viruses. It is also used in herbal remedies to relieve chest congestion, bronchitis, and chronic cough.

- **Turmeric** – Frequently described as a superfood, turmeric is a golden yellow spice loaded with antioxidants and anti-inflammatory compounds. People who eat turmeric frequently have been shown to be less susceptible to cough, cold, and congestion.

In addition to eating herbs and spices like the ones listed above, there are also some other foods that can help to boost your immune system and help you get over your chronic cough faster. Here is a list of nutrients that will help to boost your immunity and examples of foods that contain those nutrients:

- **Vitamin C** – This is the most important nutrient for the immune system and you probably know that it can be found in all citrus fruits. Because the acid in citrus fruits can aggravate irritation in your throat, you may want to focus on other food sources of vitamin C which include leafy green vegetables, brussels sprouts, bell peppers, papaya, and strawberries.
- **Vitamin E** – This vitamin is a powerful antioxidant that can help to boost your immunity and fight off infections. You can find plenty of vitamin E in broccoli, spinach, nuts, seeds, and vegetable oils.
- **Vitamin B6** – This particular vitamin plays an important role in many biochemical reactions within your body and is essential for healthy immune function. Vitamin B6 can be found in chicken breast, cold-water fish, baked potatoes, chickpeas, sunflower seeds, lean beef, avocado, and spinach.
- **Vitamin A** – You can find this vitamin in colorful foods because they are rich in carotenoids – examples include sweet potatoes, carrots, pumpkin, squash, cantaloupe, lettuce, tropical fruit, and dark leafy greens. This vitamin has strong antioxidant powers.

- **Vitamin D** – This vitamin can be absorbed from sunlight as well as some foods like fatty fish, fortified orange juice, beef liver, and egg yolks. Vitamin D is essential for balanced health and healthy immunity.
- **Folic Acid** – Also known as folate, folic acid helps to support your cardiovascular and nervous systems as well as red blood cell production. You can find folate in many foods including dried beans, avocado, dark green vegetables, and lentils.
- **Iron** – This mineral helps your body transport oxygen more efficiently which improves overall function. You can find iron in beans, broccoli, kale, lean poultry, seafood, sunflower seeds, tofu, liver, and dark chocolate.
- **Selenium** – This mineral has a powerful effect on the immune system – it can even help to slow the spread of cancer. You can find selenium in broccoli, garlic, sardines, tuna, brazil nuts, brown rice, chia seeds, sunflower seeds, mushrooms, and cabbage.
- **Zinc** – Not only does zinc help to boost immunity, but it can also help to reduce inflammation in the body. Zinc can be found in foods like chickpeas, oysters, crab, poultry, whole grains, beans, nuts and red meat.

All of the foods listed above will help you to super-charge your immune system so that you can heal from your chronic cough. You should also make an effort to follow a healthier diet in general to maximize your results. Focus on lean proteins like poultry and fish as well as fresh fruits and vegetables, whole grains, nuts, seeds, and healthy fats.

3. Cough-Busting Recipes

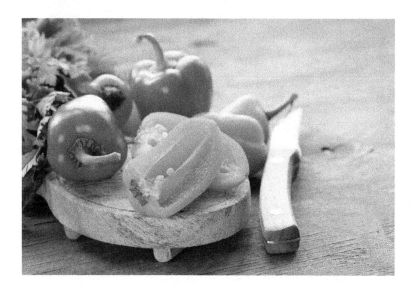

When you are suffering from persistent cough, it can sometimes be difficult to muster up the energy to cook. But eating fast food and processed foods, easy though they may be, will only make your cough last longer. If you want to kiss your cough goodbye as quickly as possible, the key is to fuel your body with healthy nutrients. In this section, you will receive a collection of recipes for teas and hot beverages as well as nutrient-rich juices and smoothies; hot and hearty soups and stews; and healthy homemade meals.

a. Teas and Hot Beverages

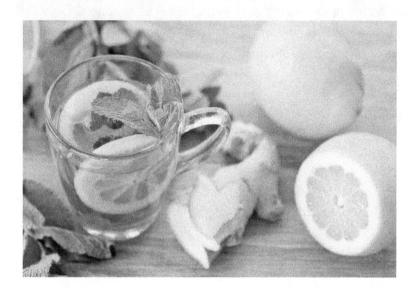

<u>Recipes Included in this Section</u>:

Anise Cinnamon Tea

Ginger Cardamom Tea

Honey Cinnamon Tea

Lemon Ginger Tea

Fresh Rosemary Tea

Cayenne Thyme Tea

Ginger Turmeric Tea

Fresh Peppermint Tea

Anise Cinnamon Tea

This recipe is incredibly easy to prepare – all you need is some anise seed and cinnamon sticks plus two bags of your favorite black tea. Feel free to adjust the lemon and honey to taste.

Servings: 2

Ingredients:

- 3 cups water
- 2 teaspoon anise seed
- 2 (2-inch) cinnamon sticks
- 1 ½ tablespoons fresh lemon juice
- 1 ½ tablespoons honey
- 2 black tea bags

Instructions:

1. Pour the water into a small saucepan.
2. Add the anise seeds and cinnamon sticks.
3. Bring the water to boil then simmer for 3 minutes.
4. Strain the mixture into a tea pot then add the lemon juice and honey.
5. Using two tea cups, place one tea bag in each cup.
6. Pour in enough hot liquid to fill the cup.
7. Let steep for 2 to 3 minutes and serve hot.

Ginger Cardamom Tea

Made with fresh ginger and cardamom, this hot tea will have you feeling better in no time. Feel free to use almond milk, coconut milk, or soy milk and sweeten to taste.

Servings: 2

Ingredients:

- 3 cups non-dairy milk
- 2 tablespoons fresh grated ginger
- 4 cardamom pods, crushed
- 4 teaspoons dried tea leaves
- Honey to taste

Instructions:

1. Pour the milk into a small saucepan and bring to a simmer.
2. Add the ginger, cardamom, and tea leaves.
3. Simmer for 5 to 6 minutes until golden brown then strain the mixture into a teapot.
4. Sweeten the tea with honey to taste and serve hot.

Honey Cinnamon Tea

All you need to make this tea is a good-quality Ceylon cinnamon stick, or two. This tea has a mild flavor and you can sweeten it to taste with honey and add lemon juice, if desired.

Servings: 2

Ingredients:

- 3 cups water
- 1 (3-inch) Ceylon cinnamon stick
- Honey, to taste

Instructions:

1. Pour the water into a small saucepan and add the cinnamon stick.
2. Bring the water to boil on medium-low heat.
3. Boil the water until the cinnamon starts to release, turning the water light brown – about 15 minutes.
4. Turn off the heat and let the cinnamon stick steep for another 15 minutes or so.

5. Remove the cinnamon stick then reheat the tea until it begins to steam.
6. Pour into teacups and sweeten with honey to taste.

Lemon Ginger Tea

Pure and simple, this lemon ginger tea is easy to make. If you prefer a stronger ginger flavor, let the tea steep longer than 10 minutes before straining it.

Servings: 2

Ingredients:

- 1 ½ tablespoons fresh grated ginger
- 2 ½ cups water
- ½ lemon, juiced
- ½ lemon, cut into wedges
- Honey to taste

Instructions:

1. Pour the water into a small saucepan and add the ginger.
2. Bring the water to boil then remove from heat.
3. Cover the saucepan and let the ginger steep for 10 minutes.
4. Strain the liquid into a teapot then add fresh lemon juice and honey to taste.
5. Pour the tea into teacups and serve hot with lemon.

Fresh Rosemary Tea

This fresh rosemary tea is very simple to make and it has a subtle aromatic flavor. You can feel free to omit the tea bag if you just want to enjoy the flavor of the fresh rosemary.

Servings: 2

Ingredients:

- 1 tablespoon fresh rosemary leaves
- 1 green tea bag
- 2 cups boiling water
- Lemon juice, to taste
- Honey, to taste

Instructions:

Chop the rosemary to release the oils then pack them into a metal tea strainer or small mesh bag.

Place the strainer in a teacup with the tea bag.

Pour in the boiling water and let steep for 5 to 10 minutes.

Remove the tea strainer and tea bag.

Add lemon juice and honey to taste, if desired.

Cayenne Thyme Tea

This tea combines the herbal power of fresh thyme with a kick of heat from the cayenne that will clear up your sinuses in a jiffy. Try inhaling some of the steam from the tea before you drink it!

Servings:

Ingredients:

- 2 tablespoons fresh chopped thyme
- 1 teaspoon fresh grated ginger
- ½ teaspoon ground turmeric
- Pinch cayenne
- 1 cup boiling water

- Lemon juice, to taste
- Honey, to taste

Instructions:

1. Place the fresh chopped thyme, ginger, turmeric, and cayenne in a tea cup.
2. Pour in the boiling water.
3. Strain the herbs and spices from the liquid.
4. Add lemon juice and honey to taste then serve hot.

Ginger Turmeric Tea

This flavorful tea blends the cough-busting power of fresh ginger with turmeric and cinnamon. If the ginger flavor is too strong for you, add more cinnamon or extra honey.

Servings: 2

Ingredients:

- 2 ½ cups water
- 1 tablespoon fresh grated ginger
- ½ teaspoon ground turmeric
- ½ teaspoon ground cinnamon
- Lemon juice, to taste
- Honey, to taste

Instructions:

1. Pour the water into a small saucepan and bring to a boil.
2. Stir in the ginger, turmeric, and cinnamon.
3. Reduce the heat and simmer on low for 10 minutes.
4. Strain the tea into two cups.
5. Add lemon juice and honey to taste and enjoy hot.

Fresh Peppermint Tea

This recipe for fresh peppermint tea couldn't be easier – all you need is fresh tea leaves and hot water. You can grow your own peppermint at home or buy a bunch at your local grocery store.

Servings:

Ingredients:

- 8 fresh peppermint leaves, torn
- 1 cup boiling water
- Honey, to taste

Instructions:

1. Place your fresh tea leaves in a teacup.
2. Pour in the boiling water and let it steep for 5 minutes.
3. Sweeten with honey to taste, if desired, and enjoy hot.

b. Nutrient-Rich Juices and Smoothies

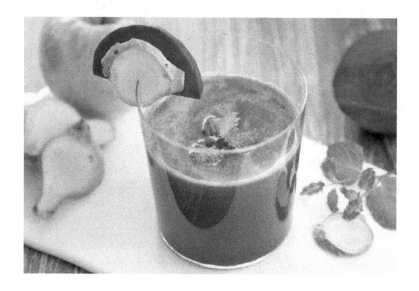

<u>Recipes Included in this Section</u>:

Watermelon Mint Smoothie

Strawberry Oatmeal Smoothie

Blackberry Red Cabbage Smoothie

Sweet Kiwi Kale Smoothie

Tropical Fruit and Greens Smoothie

Mango Coconut Smoothie

Triple Berry Spinach Smoothie

Kale Celery Apple Smoothie

Strawberry Pineapple Smoothie

Blueberry Green Smoothie

Carrot Cabbage Cucumber Juice

Spinach Kale Pear Juice

Beets and Greens Juice

Carrot Apple Ginger Juice

Spiced Sweet Potato Juice

Kale Apple Broccoli Juice

Pineapple Celery Kale Juice

Spinach Cucumber Lemonade

Broccoli Apple Juice

Cantaloupe Asparagus Juice

Watermelon Mint Smoothie

This fresh and fruity smoothie is naturally sweet and just slushy enough to be refreshing. It also has a hint of mint flavor!

Servings: 1 to 2

Ingredients:

- 2 cups fresh chopped watermelon
- 2 cups baby spinach
- 2 cups frozen pineapple
- ¼ cup fresh mint leaves
- ½ fresh lime, juiced

Instructions:

1. Combine the watermelon and spinach in a blender.
2. Add the lime juice and pulse several times to combine.
3. Blend for 10 seconds then add the remaining ingredients.
4. Pulse several times then blend for 20 to 30 seconds until the smoothie is well combined.
5. Pour the smoothie into a glass and enjoy immediately.

Strawberry Oatmeal Smoothie

Thick and creamy, this strawberry oatmeal smoothie would make a great breakfast to-go. It has whole grains for all-day energy and strawberries for natural sweetness.

Servings: 1 to 2

Ingredients:

- 2 cups unsweetened oat milk
- 1 ½ cups frozen sliced strawberries

- ¼ cup old-fashioned oats
- 1 tablespoon natural almond butter
- 1 teaspoon honey

Instructions:

1. Combine the unsweetened oat milk and strawberries in a high-speed blender.
2. Add the oats and pulse several times to combine.
3. Blend for 10 seconds then add the remaining ingredients.
4. Pulse several times then blend for 20 to 30 seconds until the smoothie is well combined.
5. Pour the smoothie into a glass and enjoy immediately.

Blackberry Red Cabbage Smoothie

This blackberry and red cabbage smoothie is absolutely packed with healthy nutrients and it tastes so sweet that you can't even tell it's good for you!

Servings: 1 to 2

Ingredients:

- 2 cups chopped red cabbage
- 1 ½ cups frozen blackberries
- 1 cup baby spinach
- 1 cup unsweetened coconut milk
- ½ lemon, juiced

Instructions:

1. Combine the cabbage, spinach and coconut milk in a high-speed blender.
2. Add the lemon juice and pulse several times to combine.
3. Blend for 10 seconds then add the remaining ingredients.

4. Pulse several times then blend for 20 to 30 seconds until the smoothie is well combined.
5. Pour the smoothie into a glass and enjoy immediately.

Sweet Kiwi Kale Smoothie

Kale is a power-packed superfood that gets a sweet kick with fresh kiwi, apple, and honey in this healthy smoothie recipe.

Servings: 1 to 2

Ingredients:

- 2 cups fresh chopped kale
- 1 medium apple, cored and chopped
- 2 ripe kiwis, peeled and sliced
- 1 ½ cups coconut water
- ½ cup ice cubes
- 1 teaspoon fresh grated ginger
- 1 teaspoon honey

Instructions:

1. Combine the kale and coconut water in a blender.
2. Add the ginger and honey then pulse several times to combine.
3. Blend for 10 seconds then add the remaining ingredients.
4. Pulse several times then blend for 20 to 30 seconds until the smoothie is well combined.
5. Pour the smoothie into a glass and enjoy immediately.

Tropical Fruit and Greens Smoothie

Tropical fruits aren't just sweet, they are also loaded with vitamins to help boost your immunity. In this smoothie recipe, they are paired with the nutritional power of fresh spinach.

Servings: 1 to 2

Ingredients:

- 2 cups baby spinach
- 1 cup frozen pineapple chunks
- ½ cup frozen papaya chunks
- 2 ripe kiwis, peeled and sliced
- 1 ½ cups coconut water
- 1 teaspoon honey
- ½ teaspoon fresh grated ginger

Instructions:

1. Combine the spinach and coconut water in a blender.
2. Add the kiwi and pulse several times to combine.
3. Blend for 10 seconds then add the remaining ingredients.
4. Pulse several times then blend for 20 to 30 seconds until the smoothie is well combined.
5. Pour the smoothie into a glass and enjoy immediately.

Pineapple Coconut Smoothie

This smoothie recipe certainly has a tropical vibe with the flavors of pineapple and coconut – you won't even notice the kale but you'll still reap the nutritional benefits!

Servings: 1 to 2

Ingredients:

- 2 cups frozen chopped pineapple

- 1 ½ cups chopped kale
- 1 cup unsweetened coconut milk
- ½ lemon, juiced

Instructions:

1. Combine the kale and coconut milk in a blender.
2. Add the lemon juice and pulse several times to combine.
3. Blend for 10 seconds then add the remaining ingredients.
4. Pulse several times then blend for 20 to 30 seconds until the smoothie is well combined.
5. Pour the smoothie into a glass and enjoy immediately.

Triple Berry Spinach Smoothie

This sweet smoothie is loaded with berries for natural sweetness and antioxidant power. The almond milk makes it nice and creamy while the spinach adds a boost of nutrition.

Servings: 1 to 2

Ingredients:

- 1 cup frozen sliced strawberries
- ½ cup frozen raspberries
- ½ cup frozen blueberries
- 1 cup fresh chopped spinach
- 1 ½ cups unsweetened almond milk
- 1 teaspoon honey

Instructions:

1. Combine the berries and almond milk in a blender.
2. Add the spinach and pulse several times to combine.
3. Blend for 10 seconds then add the honey.

4. Pulse several times then blend for 20 to 30 seconds until the smoothie is well combined.
5. Pour the smoothie into a glass and enjoy immediately.

Kale Celery Apple Smoothie

If you prefer your smoothies lightly sweetened, this is the recipe for you. You get all the nutritional benefits of fresh fruit and veggies with just a hint of sweetness from the honey.

Servings: 1 to 2

Ingredients:

- 1 ½ cups fresh chopped kale
- 1 medium apple, cored and chopped
- 1 stalk celery, sliced
- 1 ½ cups unsweetened apple juice
- 1 teaspoon honey

Instructions:

1. Combine the kale and apple juice in a high-speed blender.
2. Add the apple juice and pulse several times to combine.
3. Blend for 10 seconds then add the remaining ingredients.
4. Pulse several times then blend for 20 to 30 seconds until the smoothie is well combined.
5. Pour the smoothie into a glass and enjoy immediately.

Strawberry Pineapple Smoothie

This smoothie recipe couldn't be simpler – just throw together two of your favorite fruits (strawberries and pineapples) with some almond milk and a drizzle of honey.

Servings: 1 to 2

Ingredients:

- 1 ½ cups frozen sliced strawberries
- 1 cup frozen pineapple
- 1 cup unsweetened almond milk
- 1 tablespoon honey

Instructions:

1. Combine the strawberries and almond milk in a high-speed blender.
2. Add the pineapple and pulse several times to combine.
3. Blend for 10 seconds then add the honey.
4. Pulse several times then blend for 20 to 30 seconds until the smoothie is well combined.
5. Pour the smoothie into a glass and enjoy immediately.

Blueberry Green Smoothie

Made with both spinach and kale, this nutrient-rich smoothie will boost your immunity and kick your cough to the curb. But all you'll be tasting is the sweet blueberries and a hint of coconut.

Servings: 1 to 2

Ingredients:

- 1 ½ cups frozen blueberries
- 1 cup fresh chopped spinach
- 1 cup fresh chopped kale
- ½ medium apple, cored and chopped
- 1 cup coconut water
- 1 tablespoon honey

Instructions:

1. Combine the spinach, kale and coconut water in a high-speed blender.
2. Add the blueberries and pulse several times to combine.
3. Blend for 10 seconds then add the honey.
4. Pulse several times then blend for 20 to 30 seconds until the smoothie is well combined.
5. Pour the smoothie into a glass and enjoy immediately.

Carrot Cabbage Cucumber Juice

This tasty juice is made with the three "C"'s – carrots, cabbage, and cucumber. You'll love its fresh flavor.

Servings: 1 to 2

Ingredients:

- 2 large carrots
- 1 cup chopped cabbage
- 1 medium cucumber
- ½ bunch fresh cilantro

Instructions:

1. Place a large glass or container under the spout of your juicer.
2. Clean your ingredients then chop or slice them to fit into the juicer.
3. Feed your ingredients into the juicer in the order listed.
4. Open the juicer and scoop out the pulp.
5. Feed the pulp back through the juicer a second time.
6. Stir your juice well then enjoy immediately.

Spinach Kale Pear Juice

In addition to being loaded with nutrients, both spinach and kale are naturally low in calories, as is celery. This low-calorie juice is lightly sweetened with pear.

Servings: 1 to 2

Ingredients:

- 3 large leaves fresh kale
- ½ bunch fresh spinach
- 2 medium pears
- 1 stalk celery

Instructions:

1. Place a large glass or container under the spout of your juicer.
2. Clean your ingredients then chop or slice them to fit into the juicer.
3. Feed your ingredients into the juicer in the order listed.
4. Open the juicer and scoop out the pulp.
5. Feed the pulp back through the juicer a second time.
6. Stir your juice well then enjoy immediately.

Beets and Greens Juice

Beets have a unique flavor and they are packed with powerful vitamins and minerals. This juice also contains fresh spinach and kale as well as half a bunch of parsley.

Servings: 1 to 2

Ingredients:

- 2 cups fresh beet greens

- 1 small beet
- 2 leaves fresh kale
- 1 handful fresh spinach
- ½ bunch fresh parsley

Instructions:

1. Place a large glass or container under the spout of your juicer.
2. Clean your ingredients then chop or slice them to fit into the juicer.
3. Feed your ingredients into the juicer in the order listed.
4. Open the juicer and scoop out the pulp.
5. Feed the pulp back through the juicer a second time.
6. Stir your juice well then enjoy immediately.

Carrot Apple Ginger Juice

With carrots and apple as the main ingredients, this fresh juice has a naturally sweet flavor that pairs well with the spiced flavor of fresh ginger.

Servings: 1 to 2

Ingredients:

- 4 large leaves Swiss chard
- 1 handful fresh spinach
- 2 large carrots
- 1 medium apple
- 1 inch fresh ginger

Instructions:

1. Place a large glass or container under the spout of your juicer.
2. Clean your ingredients then chop or slice them to fit into the juicer.
3. Feed your ingredients into the juicer in the order listed.
4. Open the juicer and scoop out the pulp.
5. Feed the pulp back through the juicer a second time.
6. Stir your juice well then enjoy immediately.

Spiced Sweet Potato Juice

Sweet potatoes are not the first ingredient you might think of juicing but they combine well with high-moisture ingredients like celery and cucumber.

Servings: 1 to 2

Ingredients:

*   3 stalks celery
*   1 medium sweet potato
*   1 small cucumber
*   1 inch fresh ginger

Instructions:

1. Place a large glass under the spout of your juicer.
2. Clean your ingredients then chop or slice them to fit into the juicer.
3. Feed your ingredients into the juicer in the order listed.
4. Open the juicer and scoop out the pulp.
5. Feed the pulp back through the juicer a second time.
6. Stir your juice well then enjoy immediately.

Kale Apple Broccoli Juice

This recipe contains all green ingredients but don't worry, it has just enough sweetness from the apple to make it easy to drink.

Servings: 1 to 2

Ingredients:

- 4 large leaves kale
- 2 large ripe green apples
- 1 small head broccoli
- 1 small cucumber

Instructions:

1. Place a large glass or container under the spout of your juicer.
2. Clean your ingredients then chop or slice them to fit into the juicer.
3. Feed your ingredients into the juicer in the order listed.
4. Open the juicer and scoop out the pulp.
5. Feed the pulp back through the juicer a second time.
6. Stir your juice well then enjoy immediately.

Pineapple Celery Kale Juice

If you are looking for a hint of tropical flavor, give this pineapple celery kale juice a try. You can always stir in a splash of coconut water if you want a little more of a tropical kick.

Servings: 1 to 2

Ingredients:

- 3 large stalks celery

- ½ bunch fresh kale
- ½ ripe pineapple

Instructions:

1. Place a large glass or container under the spout of your juicer.
2. Clean your ingredients then chop or slice them to fit into the juicer.
3. Feed your ingredients into the juicer in the order listed.
4. Open the juicer and scoop out the pulp.
5. Feed the pulp back through the juicer a second time.
6. Stir your juice well then enjoy immediately.

Spinach Cucumber Lemonade

Who said lemonade couldn't be healthy? This spinach cucumber lemonade certainly is! It's like nothing you've ever had before.

Servings: 1 to 2

Ingredients:

- ½ bunch Swiss chard
- ½ bunch fresh spinach
- 1 medium cucumber
- 1 lemon, peeled

Instructions:

1. Place a large glass or container under the spout of your juicer.
2. Clean your ingredients then chop or slice them to fit into the juicer.
3. Feed your ingredients into the juicer in the order listed.

4. Open the juicer and scoop out the pulp.
5. Feed the pulp back through the juicer a second time.
6. Stir your juice well then enjoy immediately.

Broccoli Apple Juice

This power-packed juice is loaded with dark green ingredients so you can count on it being rich in nutrients. Throw in an extra apple if you need it to be a little sweeter.

Servings: 1 to 2

Ingredients:

- 1 medium head broccoli
- 1 handful fresh spinach
- 1 ripe apple

Instructions:

1. Place a large glass or container under the spout of your juicer.
2. Clean your ingredients then chop or slice them to fit into the juicer.
3. Feed your ingredients into the juicer in the order listed.
4. Open the juicer and scoop out the pulp.
5. Feed the pulp back through the juicer a second time.
6. Stir your juice well then enjoy immediately.

Cantaloupe Asparagus Juice

Fresh cantaloupe has a subtle flavor that pairs well with fresh asparagus, kale and celery in this tasty green juice.

Servings: 1 to 2

Ingredients:

- ½ medium ripe cantaloupe
- 3 large kale leaves
- ½ bunch fresh asparagus
- 1 stalk celery

Instructions:

1. Place a large glass or container under the spout of your juicer.
2. Clean your ingredients then chop or slice them to fit into the juicer.
3. Feed your ingredients into the juicer in the order listed.
4. Open the juicer and scoop out the pulp.
5. Feed the pulp back through the juicer a second time.
6. Stir your juice well then enjoy immediately.

c. Hot and Hearty Soups and Stews

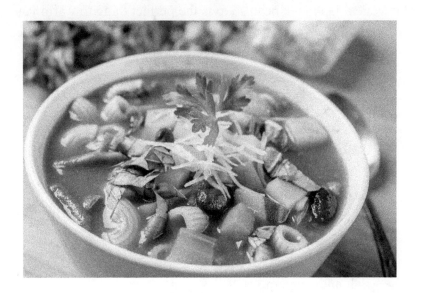

Recipes Included in this Section:

Vegetarian Black Bean Soup

Hearty Lamb and Vegetable Stew

Creamy Potato Leek Soup

Quick Beef and Barley Stew

Curried Butternut Squash Soup

Vegetable and White Bean Stew

Smoked Ham and Lentil Soup

Mediterranean Chickpea Stew

Easy Chicken and Vegetable Soup

Vegetarian Black Bean Soup

This vegetarian black bean soup is the perfect thing to warm your body and soothe your throat when you have a cough. It is studded with tender black beans and flavored with garlic and cumin.

Servings: 4 to 6

Ingredients:

- 2 tablespoons olive oil
- 2 large carrots, peeled and chopped
- 1 medium red onion, chopped
- 3 cloves minced garlic
- 1 medium bay leaf
- 2 teaspoons ground cumin
- Salt and pepper to taste
- 2 (15-ounce) cans black beans, rinsed and drained
- 1 (14-ounce) can diced tomatoes
- 4 cups vegetable or chicken broth
- ¼ cup fresh chopped cilantro, divided

Instructions:

1. Heat the oil in a Dutch oven over medium heat until hot.
2. Add the carrots and cook for 5 minutes then stir in the onions and garlic and cook for another 5 minutes.
3. Stir in the bay leaf and cumin, season with salt and pepper.
4. Pour in the beans, tomatoes, and broth then bring the mixture to a boil.
5. Reduce heat and simmer for 10 minutes then stir in 2 tablespoons of cilantro.
6. Spoon the soup into bowls and serve hot, garnished with fresh cilantro and green onions.

Hearty Lamb and Vegetable Stew

This hot and hearty lamb and vegetable stew is protein-packed and loaded with healthy nutrients. Feel free to adjust the recipe, using whatever vegetables you prefer or those you have handy.

Servings: 4 to 6

Ingredients:

- 2 pounds boneless lamb, cut into chunks
- Salt and pepper to taste
- ¼ cup all-purpose flour
- 2 tablespoons olive oil
- 1 ½ cups water
- 1 cup dry white wine
- 2 sprigs fresh thyme
- 2 sprigs fresh rosemary
- 2 cups sliced carrots
- 1 ½ cups chopped sweet potato
- 1 ½ cups chopped red potato
- 1 cup frozen peas

Instructions:

1. Season the lamb with salt and pepper to taste then toss with the flour in a large bowl.
2. Heat the oil in a Dutch oven over medium-high heat.
3. Add the lamb and cook until it is evenly browned.
4. Pour in the water and wine then add the fresh herbs.
5. Stir well then bring the mixture to boil.
6. Reduce heat and simmer, covered, for 1 hour.
7. Add the carrots, sweet potatoes, and red potatoes then cover and simmer for 45 minutes until tender.
8. Stir in the peas then cook for 5 minutes, uncovered.

9. Remove from heat and discard the herb stems then spoon into bowls and serve hot.

Creamy Potato Leek Soup

Loaded with the flavor of fresh leeks and gold potatoes, this creamy soup will go down easy. If you don't have an immersion blender, you can puree the soup in batches in a blender.

Servings: 4 to 6

Ingredients:

- 2 tablespoons olive oil
- 4 small leeks, sliced (white and light green parts only)
- 1 medium yellow onion, chopped
- 3 cloves minced garlic
- 2 large Yukon gold potatoes, peeled and chopped
- 4 cups vegetable or chicken broth
- 1 medium bay leaf
- 2 cups unsweetened almond milk
- Salt and pepper to taste

Instructions:

1. Heat the oil in a Dutch oven over medium-high heat.
2. Add the leeks, onion and garlic and cook for 7 minutes or until the onions are browned.
3. Stir in the potatoes, broth, and bay leaf then bring to a boil.
4. Reduce heat and simmer on medium-low, covered, for 35 minutes.
5. Stir in the almond milk then simmer for another 5 minutes.
6. Remove from heat and discard the bay leaf then puree the soup using an immersion blender.

7. Season with salt and pepper to taste then serve hot.

Quick Beef and Barley Stew

Lean beef and tender barley pair perfectly in this easy stew. But what really makes this stew delicious is all of those fresh herbs.

Servings: 4 to 6

Ingredients:

- 1 pound boneless beef sirloin, cut into chunks
- Salt and pepper to taste
- ¼ cup all-purpose flour
- 2 tablespoons olive oil
- 1 medium yellow onion, chopped
- 3 cloves minced garlic
- 3 cups beef broth
- 3 cups water
- 2 large carrots, peeled and chopped
- 2 stalks celery, sliced
- ¾ cup pearled barley, uncooked
- 4 sprigs fresh parsley
- 2 sprigs fresh rosemary
- 2 sprigs fresh thyme
- 2 leaves fresh basil

Instructions:

1. Season the beef with salt and pepper then toss with the flour in a large bowl until coated.
2. Heat the oil in a Dutch oven over medium-high heat.
3. Stir in the onion and cook for 5 minutes until lightly browned.

4. Add the garlic and cook for 1 minute then remove the onion and garlic to a bowl.
5. Reheat the pot with more oil and add the beef - cook until it is evenly browned on all sides.
6. Pour in the broth and water then stir in the cooked onions and garlic.
7. Stir in the carrots, celery and barley then season with salt and pepper to taste.
8. Tie together the herbs then add to the pot.
9. Bring the mixture to boil then simmer, uncovered, for 30 minutes until the barley is tender.
10. Remove the fresh herbs then spoon the stew into bowls.

Curried Butternut Squash Soup

The perfect fall recipe, this curried butternut squash soup is a snap to prepare. If you don't have butternut squash, feel free to try it with acorn squash or your favorite winter squash.

Servings: 4 to 6

Ingredients:

- 2 tablespoons olive oil
- 1 medium yellow onion, chopped
- ½ cup chopped carrot
- ½ cup diced celery
- 4 cups fresh chopped butternut squash
- 4 cups chicken broth or vegetable broth
- ½ teaspoon fresh chopped thyme
- ½ teaspoon curry powder
- Salt and pepper to taste

Instructions:

1. Heat the oil in a Dutch oven over medium-high heat.
2. Add the onion, carrot and celery then cook for 3 to 4 minutes until lightly browned.
3. Stir in the butternut squash along with the chicken broth thyme, and curry powder.
4. Season with salt and pepper then stir well and bring the mixture to boil.
5. Reduce heat and simmer, uncovered, for 30 minutes until the squash is tender.
6. Remove from heat and puree using an immersion blender.
7. Spoon into bowls and serve with a drizzle of coconut milk or almond milk to serve.

Vegetable and White Bean Stew

Loaded to the brim with tender vegetables, this hearty stew will have you feeling better in no time. Feel free to swap out the white beans for whatever type of bean you prefer.

Servings: 4 to 6

Ingredients:

- 2 cups white cannellini beans, dried
- Water, as needed
- 1 large onion, chopped
- 4 medium carrots, peeled and chopped
- 2 stalks celery, sliced
- 2 medium turnips, peeled and sliced
- 2 medium parsnips, peeled and sliced
- 1 teaspoon fresh chopped thyme
- 1 teaspoon fresh chopped rosemary
- Pinch ground cloves

- Salt and pepper to taste
- 2 to 3 cups fresh chopped kale

Instructions:

1. Place the beans in a bowl then cover with water and let soak overnight.
2. Drain and rinse the beans then place them in a large Dutch oven.
3. Add water to cover the beans by 2 inches then heat over medium-high heat until boiling.
4. Skim off the foam then add the onion, carrots, celery, turnips, parsnips, herbs and spices to the pot.
5. Reduce heat and simmer on medium-low, covered, for about 45 minutes until the beans are tender.
6. Discard the bay leaf then season with salt and pepper.
7. Stir in the kale and cook until just wilted then spoon the stew into bowls and serve hot.

Smoked Ham and Lentil Soup

Tender lentils and smoked ham are the perfect match in this delicious soup. If you are feeling adventurous, you could even try it with dried split peas instead of lentils!

Servings: 6 to 8

Ingredients:

- 2 tablespoons olive oil
- 1 large yellow onion, chopped
- 2 small carrots, peeled and chopped
- 2 stalks celery, chopped
- 3 cloves minced garlic

- 1 cup dried green lentils
- 1 (14-ounce) can diced tomatoes
- 1 cup diced smoked ham
- 1 medium ham bone
- 8 cups chicken broth
- 1 teaspoon fresh chopped thyme
- 1 teaspoon fresh chopped rosemary
- 1 teaspoon fresh chopped tarragon
- 1 medium bay leaf
- Salt and pepper to taste

Instructions:

1. Heat the oil in a Dutch oven over medium-high heat.
2. Add the onions, carrots, celery and garlic then cook for 5 to 6 minutes until the onions are translucent.
3. Stir in the lentils, tomatoes and ham then add the ham bone.
4. Pour in the broth then stir in the herbs and bring to a boil.
5. Reduce heat and simmer, covered, for 25 to 30 minutes.
6. Stir well then simmer for another 30 minutes or until the lentils are tender – add more broth if needed.
7. Remove from heat and discard the bay leaf and ham bone.
8. Adjust seasoning to taste then spoon into bowls to serve.

Mediterranean Chickpea Stew

This recipe is incredibly simple but it is not lacking in flavor. Studded with tender chickpeas and flavored with fresh garlic, you are going to love this Mediterranean-style stew.

Servings: 4 to 6

Ingredients:

- 2 tablespoons olive oil
- 1 large yellow onion, chopped
- 3 cloves minced garlic
- 1 medium red pepper, cored and chopped
- 2 large zucchini, chopped
- 2 (14-ounce) cans crushed tomatoes
- 1 (15-ounce) can chickpeas, rinsed and drained
- Salt and pepper to taste

Instructions:

1. Heat the oil in a Dutch oven over medium-high heat.
2. Add the onions and garlic and cook for 5 to 6 minutes until the onions are translucent.
3. Stir in the red peppers and cook for 5 minutes, then add the zucchini and cook for 12 to 15 minutes.
4. Add the tomatoes, crushing them with the back of a wooden spoon, then bring to a simmer.
5. Cook on medium-low heat for 20 minutes then stir in the chickpeas.
6. Let the soup simmer for another 5 minutes then season with salt and pepper to taste and serve hot.

Easy Chicken and Vegetable Soup

Nothing soothes a sore throat like homemade chicken and vegetable soup. Don't be afraid to load this one up with extra veggies if you want to make it a little more filling!

Servings: 6 to 8

Ingredients:

- 2 tablespoons olive oil

- 3 cloves minced garlic
- 1 teaspoon fresh chopped oregano
- 1 ¼ cups frozen corn kernels
- 1 small red pepper, chopped
- 1 small poblano pepper, chopped
- 4 cups chicken broth or vegetable broth
- ½ cup tomato sauce
- Salt and pepper to taste
- ½ small zucchini, sliced
- ½ small summer squash, sliced
- ¼ cup fresh chopped basil
- ½ teaspoon fresh chopped rosemary
- ¼ teaspoon fresh chopped tarragon
- 2 green onions, sliced thin

Instructions:

1. Heat the oil in a Dutch oven over medium-high heat.
2. Add the garlic cloves and oregano then cook for 1 minute.
3. Stir in the corn and the peppers then cook for 3 to 4 minutes until the peppers are just starting to soften.
4. Pour in the broth and tomato sauce then stir in the chicken.
5. Season with salt and pepper to taste then stir well and bring the mixture to boil.
6. Add the zucchini and summer squash then reduce heat and simmer for 5 minutes.
7. Remove the soup from heat and stir in the fresh herbs and green onions then spoon into bowls to serve.

d. Healthy Homemade Meals for Cough

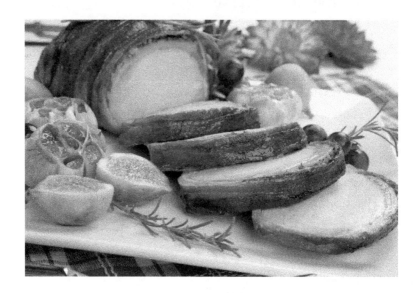

<u>Recipes Included in this Section</u>:

Herb Roasted Chicken with Veggies

Balsamic Grilled Salmon

Lemon Herb-Crusted Pork Tenderloin

Coconut Vegetable Curry

Honey Mustard Baked Chicken Tenders

Sesame-Crusted Seared Tuna

Slow-Cooker Pot Roast with Sweet Potatoes

Rosemary Thyme Roasted Lamb Chops

Herb Roasted Chicken with Veggies

If you are looking for a hot and hearty meal that takes little time to prepare, look no further than this herb roasted chicken with vegetables. You cook it all in one dish – what could be easier?

Servings: 4 to 6

Ingredients:

- 2 tablespoons olive oil
- 2 ½ pounds bone-in chicken thighs
- Salt and pepper to taste
- 2 medium sweet potatoes, chopped
- 2 large carrots, sliced
- 2 stalks celery, sliced
- 1 large onion, chopped
- 1 large head broccoli, chopped
- ¼ cup chicken broth
- 2 teaspoons fresh chopped rosemary
- 2 teaspoons fresh chopped thyme

Instructions:

1. Preheat the oven to 400°F.
2. Heat the oil in a large skillet over medium-high heat.
3. Season the chicken with salt and pepper to taste then add it to the skillet and cook until browned on all sides.
4. Meanwhile, toss the vegetables with the chicken broth, rosemary, and thyme and season with salt and pepper.
5. Spread the vegetable mixture in a large glass baking dish then place the chicken thighs skin-side down on top.
6. Bake the chicken and veggies for 30 minutes then turn the chicken and cook for another 25 to 30 minutes until the juices run clear.

7. Serve the chicken hot with the vegetables on the side.

Balsamic Grilled Salmon

This balsamic grilled salmon is very easy to prepare and it is sure to pair well with your favorite side dish. So heat up the grill, buy some fresh fish at the market, and grill away!

Servings: 4

Ingredients:

- ¼ cup fresh lemon juice
- 2 tablespoons olive oil
- 2 tablespoons balsamic vinegar
- 1 teaspoon Dijon mustard
- 4 (6-ounce) boneless salmon fillets
- Salt and pepper to taste

Instructions:

1. Whisk together the lemon juice, oil, balsamic vinegar and mustard in a shallow dish.
2. Season the salmon fillets with salt and pepper to taste then place them in the dish.
3. Turn to coat then cover and chill for at least 30 minutes.
4. Preheat the grill to medium-high heat and brush the grates with olive oil.
5. Place the fillets on the grill and cook for 4 minutes per side, brushing occasionally with extra marinade.

Lemon Herb-Crusted Pork Tenderloin

Not only is this recipe incredibly simple to prepare, but it is also easy to multiply. If you are throwing a dinner party, just double or triple the recipe so everyone can enjoy it!

Servings: 6 to 8

Ingredients:

- 2 tablespoons olive oil
- 2 teaspoons minced garlic
- 2 teaspoons fresh grated ginger
- 1 teaspoon fresh chopped rosemary
- 1 teaspoon fresh chopped thyme
- 1 teaspoon fresh chopped oregano
- Salt and pepper to taste
- 2 (1-pound) boneless pork tenderloins

Instructions:

1. Preheat the oven to 400°F and line a roasting pan with foil.
2. Place the oil in a small bowl then add the garlic and ginger – season with salt and pepper.
3. Mash the garlic and ginger with a fork to form a sort of paste.
4. Stir in the lemon juice and herbs then rub the mixture all over the pork tenderloin.
5. Place the tenderloin in the roasting pan and surround it with the sliced onions.
6. Bake for 25 to 35 minutes until the internal temperature reads 160°F.
7. Remove the tenderloin to a cutting board and cover loosely with foil.
8. Let the tenderloin rest for 10 minutes, slice to serve.

Coconut Vegetable Curry

Not every meal has to include meat and this coconut vegetable curry is still hot and filling without it. Feel free to throw in some extra vegetables or add some cayenne to give it a little heat.

Servings: 4 to 6

Ingredients:

- 1 tablespoon olive oil
- 1 medium yellow onion, chopped
- 3 cloves minced garlic
- 1 tablespoon fresh grated ginger
- 2 medium carrots, peeled and chopped
- 2 small heads broccoli, chopped
- Salt and pepper to taste
- 1 tablespoon curry powder
- 2 (14-ounce) cans coconut milk
- 1 cup vegetable broth
- 1 medium tomato, diced

Instructions:

1. Heat the oil in a deep skillet over medium heat.
2. Add the onion and cook for 3 minutes then stir in the garlic and ginger and cook for another 2 minutes.
3. Stir in the carrots and broccoli then season with salt and pepper to taste.
4. Cook the vegetables until they begin to soften, about 5 minutes.
5. Stir in the curry powder along with the coconut milk and vegetable stock.
6. Bring to a boil then reduce heat and simmer for 10 to 15 minutes until thickened.

7. Stir in the tomatoes and cook for 5 minutes then serve hot.

Honey Mustard Baked Chicken Tenders

Skip the fast food and go straight for these honey mustard baked chicken tenders. This recipe is incredibly easy to prepare – just make the sauce then pour it over the chicken and bake it!

Servings: 5 to 6

Ingredients:

- ½ cup honey
- 4 tablespoons Dijon mustard
- 4 tablespoons whole grain mustard
- ½ tablespoon olive oil
- 1 medium yellow onion, chopped
- 3 cloves minced garlic
- 2 ½ pounds boneless skinless chicken tenderloins
- Salt and pepper to taste

Instructions:

1. Preheat the oven to 400°F.
2. Whisk together the honey, mustards, olive oil and salt.
3. Grease a large ovenproof skillet and heat it over medium heat.
4. Add the onions and cook for 5 minutes until tender then add the garlic and cook 1 minute more.
5. Place the chicken tenderloins in the skillet then season with salt and pepper.
6. Pour the honey mustard sauce over the chicken then transfer the skillet to the oven.
7. Bake, covered with foil, for 20 minutes.

8. Remove the foil and baste the chicken then bake for another 20 to 30 minutes uncovered until cooked through.

Sesame-Crusted Seared Tuna

If you enjoy fresh fish, you'll love this sesame-crusted seared tuna. It is so delicious that you'll feel like you're dining at a restaurant but it only takes a few minutes to prepare!

Servings: 4

Ingredients:

- 4 (6-ounce) ahi tuna steaks
- Salt and pepper to taste
- ¼ cup black sesame seeds
- ¼ cup white sesame seeds
- 2 tablespoons olive oil

Instructions:

1. Season the tuna steaks with salt and pepper.
2. Combine the black and white sesame seeds in a shallow dish then press the steaks into them, coating all sides.
3. Heat the oil in a large skillet over high heat until smoking.
4. Add the tuna steaks and cook for 1 minute until seared.
5. Turn the steaks and cook for another minute.
6. Transfer the steaks to a cutting board and slice thin.

Slow-Cooker Pot Roast with Sweet Potatoes

The slow cooker is a wonderful appliance to have around – all you have to do is prepare your ingredients then throw them together and let them cook! You'll come home to a hot meal.

Servings: 4 to 6

Ingredients:

- 2 tablespoons olive oil
- 2 pounds boneless beef chuck roast
- Salt and pepper to taste
- 2 medium onions, sliced thin
- 3 large sweet potatoes, peeled and cut into chunks
- 1 cup beef broth
- 1 teaspoon fresh chopped rosemary
- 1 ½ tablespoons cornstarch
- 2 tablespoons cold water

Instructions:

1. Heat the oil in a large skillet over medium-high heat.
2. Season the pot roast with salt and pepper then add to the skillet and brown on all sides.
3. Combine the onions and chopped sweet potatoes in the slow cooker then place the roast on top.
4. Whisk together the remaining ingredients aside from the cornstarch and water then pour into the slow cooker.
5. Cover and cook on low heat for 7 to 8 hours or on high heat for 4 to 5 hours.
6. Remove the roast to a cutting board and tent loosely with foil.
7. Spoon out the vegetables into a serving bowl.
8. Whisk together the cornstarch and water then stir in the juices in the slow cooker.
9. Cook on low heat for 5 minutes or until thickened.
10. Cut the roast into chunks and serve with the sweet potatoes and gravy.

Rosemary Thyme Roasted Lamb Chops

There is no better way to enjoy fresh herbs than mashed with garlic and spread over some tasty lamb chops. So head to your garden, cut some herbs, and get cooking!

Servings: 4

Ingredients:

- 2 pounds thick lamb chops
- Salt and pepper to taste
- ¼ cup olive oil
- 5 cloves minced garlic
- 1 ½ tablespoons fresh chopped rosemary
- 2 teaspoons fresh chopped thyme

Instructions:

- Season the lamb chops to taste with salt and pepper.
- Combine the olive oil, garlic, and herbs and mash into a paste with a fork.
- Rub the paste into the lamb chops on both sides then let them rest for 30 minutes.
- Generously grease a skillet and heat it over medium-high heat until hot.
- Add the lamb chops and cook for 2 minutes then flip and cook for 3 to 3 ½ minutes until cooked to the desired level.

Chapter 7: How Can You Help?

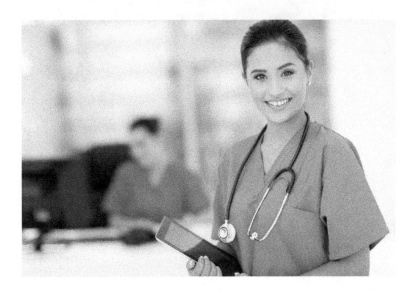

If you've ever fallen victim to chronic cough, you know how unpleasant it can be and you are not alone! Countless individuals struggle with chronic cough and dry cough each and every year, some of them never receive treatment. But even though millions suffer with cough each year, each new year also brings new medical research. In this chapter, you'll receive an overview of some new research and clinical studies that are being conducted about chronic cough and dry cough. You'll also receive tips for supporting a loved one suffering from chronic cough or dry cough.

1. Research and Studies Being Conducted

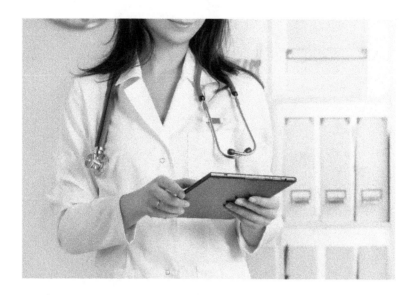

Clinical researchers are always engaging in medical studies to learn more about various health problems and how they can be relieved. <u>Below you will find a list of some of the many studies that have been recently completed or are currently underway that involve chronic cough or dry cough</u>:

- *The Use of Capsaicin Challenge for Diagnosis, Monitoring and Follow-Up of Chronic Cough.* Tel-Aviv Sourasky Medical Center. March 2013.

- *Lidocaine: Effect of Lidocaine in Chronic Cough.* University Hospital of South Manchester NHS Foundation Trust. November 2010.

- *Surgery in Chronic Cough GERD Related.* University of Bologna. July 2013.

- *A Study to Identify and Characterize Bacteria Causing Chronic Cough Among Children in United Kingdom.* GlaxoSmithKline. February 2011.

- *Impact of Gastroesophageal Reflux and Aspiration on Airway Inflammation and Microbiome in Children with Chronic Cough.* New York University School of Medicine. June 2016.

- *Treatment of Chronic Cough in Idiopathic Pulmonary Fibrosis with Thalidomide.* Johns Hopkins University. January 2008.

- *Iron Repletion in Chronic Cough and Iron Deficiency.* University of Turin, Italy. December 2011.

- *Sputum and Plasma Levels of Nociceptin and Substance P in Patients with Asthma, COPD and Chronic Cough.* National Taiwan University Hospital. September 2005.

- *Neurophysiology and Pharmacology of Cough Reflex Hypersensitivity.* University of Manchester. March 2009.

- *Predictive Factors in Response to Inhaled Corticoids in Chronic Cough.* Universite Catholique de Louvain. March 2016.

- *Cough Responses to Tussive Agents in Health and Disease.* University Hospital of South Manchester NHS Foundation Trust. February 2011.

- *An Investigation into the Mechanism of Inhalation Cough Challenge*. Hull and East Yorkshire Hospitals NHS Trust. December 2013.

- *Exhaled Breath Condensate pH in Patients with Cough Caused by Gastroesophageal Reflux*. University of Massachusetts. March 2007.

- *Clinical Assessment of Patients with Chronic Obstructive Pulmonary Disease (COPD) and/or Chronic Heart Failure (CHF)*. University of Modena and Reggio Emilia. April 2010.

- *Cough Reflex Sensitivity and Bronchial Hyper-Responsiveness*. Mayo Clinic. January 2013.

2. Tips for Supporting a Family Member

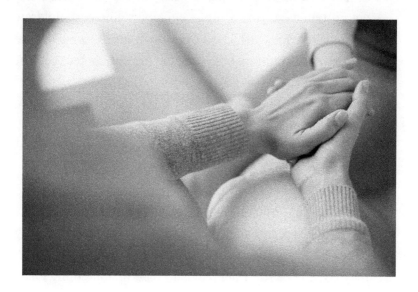

When a member of your family is sick it can be painful to watch them suffer. You may not be able to cure them, but there are things you can do to help them through it. Here are some simple things you can do to support a family member or friend who is suffering from chronic cough or dry cough:

- Be available to run minor errands for the individual so that they can stay home and rest – you can pick up prescriptions, go to the grocery store, and do other tasks.
- Make sure that your loved one is drinking plenty of fluids. Water, clear broth, fruit juices, and unsweetened sports drinks are all good things for them to have.
- If your loved one is too sick to get out of bed, offer to help them clean up with a warm washcloth or sponge. You should also help them to change their clothes and keep their bed linens clean.

- For those who are able to eat, warm up healthy soups and other nutritious meals that are easy to eat. Make sure they get protein as well as fruits, vegetables, and carbohydrates.
- Keep an eye on your loved one's symptoms to make sure they are not getting worse – if you are concerned, call the patient's doctor and ask questions.
- Make sure that your loved one is able to breathe – some causes for chronic cough can result in breathing difficulties. It may help to prop your loved one up with pillows to keep their airway open.
- Check the person's heart beat once in a while as an indication of circulation – the longer they stay in bed, the higher the risk that they may form a blood clot.
- Keep the patient warm and comfortable and make sure that they have books or magazines to read or something else to keep them occupied when they are awake.
- Monitor the patient's medications if they are taking any. Some causes for chronic cough can also cause mental fog – you don't want your loved one to get confused about dosage and take too much medication.

If a member of your family falls ill, do everything you can to help them get well. Depending on the severity of the illness, all you may have to do is help them around the house and make sure that they stay hydrated. If you begin to worry that your loved one is getting worse, do not hesitate to call a doctor.

Chapter 8: Helpful Websites and Resources

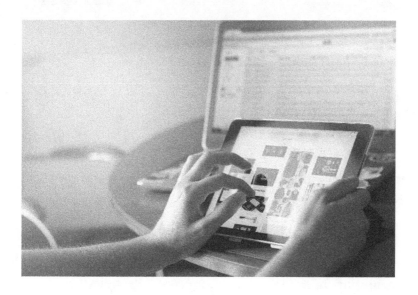

If you are suffering from chronic or dry cough, you may want to take the time to learn a little bit more about your condition and possible treatment options. In the following pages, you will find a collection of websites and other resources to help you educate yourself about the different causes for cough and about treatment options that you might consider. Each of the links provided will take you to a website where you can find additional resources about the topic listed.

Chest Foundation – Patient Education Resources.

http://www.chestnet.org/Foundation/Patient-Education-Resources/Patient-Education-Resources

National Heart, Lung, and Blood Institute – Cough Resources.

https://www.nhlbi.nih.gov/health/health-topics/topics/cough

COPD Foundation – What is COPD?

http://www.copdfoundation.org/What-is-COPD/Understanding-COPD/What-is-COPD.aspx

International Foundation for Functional Gastrointestinal Disorders – About GERD. http://www.aboutgerd.org/

American Academy of Otolaryngology – Patient Health Information. http://www.entnet.org/content/patient-health

World Health Organization – Respiratory Tract Diseases.

http://www.who.int/topics/respiratory_tract_diseases/en/

American Academy of Allergy Asthma & Immunology.

http://www.aaaai.org/conditions-and-treatments/

American Lung Association – Lung Health & Diseases.

http://www.lung.org/lung-health-and-diseases/

Index

A

B

C

Index

Index

M

N

O

Index

S

Index

Index

X

References

"5 Spices to Help with Coughs." Tuslage.
<https://tulsage.wordpress.com/2013/10/09/five-spices-to-help-with-coughs/>

"7 Immunity-Boosting Foods to Fight Colds and Flu." Daily
Burn. <http://dailyburn.com/life/health/immune-system-foods-colds-flu/>

"7 Natural Cough Remedies for Persistent & Dry Cough."
Everyday Roots. <http://everydayroots.com/cough-remedies>

"Acid Reflux (GERD) Statistics and Facts." Healthline.
<http://www.healthline.com/health/gerd/statistics>

"Anxiety Cough Symptoms, Chronic Cough and/or Nervous
Cough Symptoms." Anxiety Centre.
<http://www.anxietycentre.com/anxiety/symptoms/anxiety-cough.shtml>

"Asthma." Mayo Clinic. <http://www.mayoclinic.org/diseases-conditions/asthma/basics/definition/con-20026992>

"Chronic Cough." Mayo Clinic. <http://www.mayoclinic.org/
diseases-conditions/chronic-cough/home/ovc-20201781>

"Chronic Obstructive Pulmonary Disease (COPD)." Centers for
Disease Control and Prevention. <https://www.cdc.gov/copd/
index.html>

"COPD." Mayo Clinic. <http://www.mayoclinic.org/diseases-conditions/copd/home/ovc-20204882>

"Cough Symptoms and Treatment." Parents.com.
<http://www.parents.com/health/cough/cough/>

"Coughs, Age 12 and Older – Prevention." WebMD. <http://www.webmd.com/cold-and-flu/tc/coughs-prevention>

"Diet and Fruits for Cough." Diet Health Club. <http://www.diethealthclub.com/health-issues-and-diet/cough/diet.html>

"Dry Cough." A. Vogel. <http://www.avogel.co.uk/health/immune-system/cough/dry/>

"Dry Cough." The Health Site. <http://www.thehealthsite.com/diseases-conditions/dry-cough/001/>

"Dry Cough." WebMD. <http://www.webmd.com/cold-and-flu/tc/dry-coughs-topic-overview>

Duggal, Neel. "Is Dry Cough a Symptom of HIV?" Healthline. <http://www.healthline.com/health/hiv-aids/hiv-dry-cough#Overview1>

"Eat These Foods to Boost Your Immune System." Cleveland Clinic. <https://health.clevelandclinic.org/2015/01/eat-these-foods-to-boost-your-immune-system/>

"Flu or Cold Symptoms?" WebMD. <http://www.webmd.com/cold-and-flu/cold-guide/flu-cold-symptoms#1>

Griffin, Amanda. "What Not to Eat When You're Down with Cough and Colds." Amanda Griffin-Jacob. <http://amandagriffinjacob.com/foods-avoid-cough-cold-flu/>

Griffin, R. Morgan. "8 Reasons Your Cough is Not Improving." WebMD. <http://www.webmd.com/cold-and-flu/features/stubborn-cough#1>

"How to Take Care of a Sick Person." Hesperian Health Guides. <https://hesperian.org/wp-content/uploads/pdf/en_wtnd_2015/en_wtnd_2015_04.pdf>

References

Levine, Hallie. "7 Kinds of Cough and What They Might Mean." Health.com. <http://www.health.com/cold-flu-sinus/whats-causing-your-cough>

Mahashur, Ashok. "Chronic Dry Cough: Diagnostic and Management Approaches." *Lung India*. 2015 Jan-Feb; 32(1): 44-49. <http://www.webmd.com/cold-and-flu/features/stubborn-cough#1>

"Mechanism of a Cough." Medscape. <http://emedicine.medscape.com/article/1048560-overview#a2>

"Obstructive Sleep Apnea Explained." WebMD. <http://www.webmd.com/sleep-disorders/guide/understanding-obstructive-sleep-apnea-syndrome#1>

"Pertussis (Whooping Cough)." Centers for Disease Control and Prevention. <https://www.cdc.gov/pertussis/>

Pietrangelo, Ann. "COPD by the Numbers: Facts, Statistics, and You." Healthline. <http://www.healthline.com/health/copd/facts-statistics-infographic#1>

"Pneumonia." Mayo Clinic. <http://www.mayoclinic.org/diseases-conditions/pneumonia/home/ovc-20204676>

"That Nagging Cough." Harvard Health Publications. <http://www.health.harvard.edu/staying-healthy/that-nagging-cough>

"Types of Cough." Benylin. <https://www.benylin.co.uk/types-of-cough>

"Vocal Cord Dysfunction (VCD) or Paradoxical Vocal Fold Movement (PVFM)." American Academy of Allergy Asthma & Immunology. <http://www.aaaai.org/conditions-and-treatments/related-conditions/vocal-cord-dysfunction>

"What is COPD?" National Heart, Lung, and Blood Institute. <https://www.nhlbi.nih.gov/health/health-topics/topics/copd>

"What is Postnasal Drip?" WebMD. <http://www.webmd.com/allergies/postnasal-drip#1>

"Whooping Cough." Mayo Clinic. <http://www.mayoclinic.org/diseases-conditions/whooping-cough/basics/definition/con-20023295>

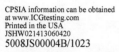
CPSIA information can be obtained
at www.ICGtesting.com
Printed in the USA
JSHW021413060420
5008JS00004B/1023